The Luckiest Unlucky Couple

The Luckiest Unlucky Couple

A Medical Love Story

Alicia C. Shepard

BLOOMSBURY ACADEMIC
NEW YORK • LONDON • OXFORD • NEW DELHI • SYDNEY

BLOOMSBURY ACADEMIC

Bloomsbury Publishing Inc, 1359 Broadway, New York, NY 10018, USA
Bloomsbury Publishing Plc, 50 Bedford Square, London, WC1B 3DP, UK
Bloomsbury Publishing Ireland, 29 Earlsfort Terrace, Dublin 2, D02 AY28, Ireland

BLOOMSBURY, BLOOMSBURY ACADEMIC and the Diana logo
are trademarks of Bloomsbury Publishing Plc

First published in the United States of America 2026

Copyright © David Marsden, 2026

Cover design: Jen Huppert Design
Cover illustration created by Tabitha Lahr
Cover images © shutterstock/LidiaKubrak; shutterstock/Prostock-studio;
shutterstock/Cristina Conti; iStock.com/Sandor Mejias Brito

All rights reserved. No part of this publication may be: i) reproduced or transmitted in any form, electronic or mechanical, including photocopying, recording or by means of any information storage or retrieval system without prior permission in writing from the publishers; or ii) used or reproduced in any way for the training, development or operation of artificial intelligence (AI) technologies, including generative AI technologies. The rights holders expressly reserve this publication from the text and data mining exception as per Article 4(3) of the Digital Single Market Directive (EU) 2019/790.

Bloomsbury Publishing Inc does not have any control over, or responsibility for, any third-party websites referred to or in this book. All internet addresses given in this book were correct at the time of going to press. The author and publisher regret any inconvenience caused if addresses have changed or sites have ceased to exist, but can accept no responsibility for any such changes.

A catalog record for this book is available from the Library of Congress.

ISBN: HB: 979-8-216-27005-8
ePDF: 979-8-216-27007-2
eBook: 979-8-216-27006-5

Typeset by Integra Software Services Pvt. Ltd.
Printed and bound in the United States of America

For product safety related questions contact productsafety@bloomsbury.com.

To find out more about our authors and books visit www.bloomsbury.com
and sign up for our newsletters.

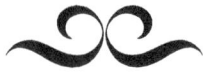

Contents

Foreword by Cutter Hodierne vii

1 One Life to Live 1

2 I Don't Have a Little White Dog 7

3 Trauma Never Leaves 15

4 Afghanistan 19

5 A Constellation of Strangers 39

6 Recovery Is a Rough Road 53

7 Reclaiming Our Lives 67

8 The Seizure That Ended the Sailing Trip 73

9 The New New Normal 85

10 My Turn 91

11 We Can Help You 103

12 The EGFR Jackpot 109

13 Losing Judy 115

14 Who Am I with Cancer? 119

15 The Grand Canyon 129

16 Scanziety 135

17 C797S and the CyberKnife 141

18 Dog No. 1 149

19 Whack the Mole 157

20 When One Person in Your Boat Is Calm 167

Epilogue by David Marsden 175
Appendix: Advice for Patients, Families, and Friends 195
About the Author 201

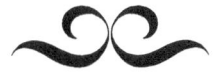

Foreword

Cutter Hodierne

For my mom, life was all about stories—finding them, chasing them, telling them. Her antenna was always up and active. Her books and articles were ambitious and diverse, winning many awards and positive reviews. But while she won acclaim for her work about other people, it was her heartfelt personal stories that were the ones I loved the most.

My mom's career was focused largely on media ethics and the journalist's process. Her books, *Woodward & Bernstein: Life in the Shadow of Watergate* and *Running Toward Danger*, which documented the harrowing stories of journalists on 9/11, and her work as NPR's ombudsman all focused on the way reporters cover news stories and the ethics employed in doing so. She was brilliant at that. But to me, stories like "Letters from Paradise," which documented our voyage across the Pacific Ocean on a sailboat with a baby (me); "Dispatches from the Love Front," her diary from Afghanistan; or her spiky *Washington Post* article "A's for Everyone," about her experience as a journalism professor with rampant grade inflation, were where her humanity and personality shone through.

My mom was resilient and courageous. She was also blunt and honest. And, for lack of a better word, *nosy*. (And I do mean that as a compliment!) She would always ask the question no one would ask, and she was interested in everyone. If she sat next to you on an airplane, she would know your whole story by the time the plane landed.

This made her an elite journalist, but it also made her a thoroughly engaged mother. She knew all the characters in my life. She knew everyone's name, their backgrounds, our connections, our battles. That to me was how she showed love. These qualities all combined to make her a fascinating woman but an even more fun person to be around. A screech to a freeway exit for an impulsive trip to a water park wasn't unusual. Nor was staying up late into the night with my friends sharing gossip. Her prying about your love life didn't embarrass you. She made you feel interesting. She made you feel seen and heard. If there was a party, she'd go. If there was a trip to take, she'd do it. If there was dancing, she'd get out on the dance floor; she was nonstop fun. She always said, "You've got to suck the marrow out of life." I felt like the luckiest kid on earth to have a mom like this—brilliant, super-fun, spontaneous, and loving.

That's what makes this so hard to write. Her absence has left a gaping hole in my heart. Her journey through love and through her medical challenges is the story we're here to share with you. She was a reporter to her core. And now she has turned that gaze onto herself. And this is her most personal story of all.

When David, my mom's husband/my stepdad, received a shocking diagnosis of stage 4 melanoma and needed emergency surgery to save his life, my mom was devastated. To manage her shock, fear, and trauma, she turned it into a story, and her curiosity went into overdrive. Learning about new cancer treatments, finding reliable sources, and connecting the dots.

The weird thing about cancer is that it forces you to become a bit of an expert in something you never wanted to know about. You become a frontline worker. Only it's your house that's on fire and now you're holding the wildly flailing hose. You have no choice but to hold on.

Through David's medical battles and then, ultimately, her own challenges with cancer, the last years of her life threw David and my mom into stormy seas. And in the valleys between big swells, my mom found her footing. My mom held on. She didn't give up on anything, especially the people she loved. She was a reporter to her core. She told us a story.

My mom's curiosity and passion for storytelling were contagious. As these awful cancers have ravaged our family, the battles have also brought us closer. She once penned an article, "Cancer Made Us a Family," about our experiences melding two families of stepkids through a medical love story. Up to this point, I was an only child. And while I wouldn't wish these experiences on anybody, in the end, my family grew, and we all came to love and support one another. This book is an example of how some of her best work was born from a bad situation, but one that led her to make profound discoveries about our human experience. To be grateful. To be present.

My grandmother used to say, "Lisa, not *everything* is a story!" But my grandmother was wrong. Story is how my mom interpreted the world and how she shared her love with all of us. So, this is her final story. And she worked on it until the final days of her life. At times, even falling asleep at the keyboard, trying to finish this before it was too late. In these pages, her voice lives on, one last chance to connect, to uncover, and to remind us all of the beauty in asking questions. Not only to others but also of ourselves.

1

One Life to Live

I brought our dog, River, to David's brain MRI. It was February 2017, and David was going in for a routine scan at a local imaging center. They wanted to make sure that a stage 2 melanoma, a purplish pea-size bump on his head, hadn't spread before he underwent surgery to remove it. I would walk River while David knocked out the MRI.

We weren't worried. The first biopsy report had been encouraging, as it "favored" a nodule over evidence of any spread. The surgeon had even reassured us he could remove the lump after we returned from a trip to Los Angeles. We were due to leave in two days.

But nothing was routine about that MRI.

When I got back to the waiting area, the doctor called David and me into a private room. He said that David, who was otherwise healthy at sixty-five, had six tumors growing in his brain—three of them grape-size. The doctor was concerned that David was in imminent danger of a seizure or stroke, so he sent us to the nearest emergency department at a local hospital in Virginia.

The neurologist's assistant at the hospital who was viewing the scans quickly let us know—*twice*—how bad things were. As she pointed out the three large tumors to David (I couldn't look), she explained that because they were on different sides of his brain, it made surgery problematic. Given the size of the tumors, she added, it was likely the cancer had spread to other parts of his body.

"Unfortunately," she said, "this is how melanoma metastasizes."

No one, I would venture, is ever prepared for a cancer diagnosis. It rocks your world in an instant. *How could this be happening?* We should've been home by now from the routine MRI, getting dinner ready, and packing for our trip to LA, excited to see David's eldest son, Ted, and my son, Cutter, as well as my favorite niece, Lydia.

Instead, David was admitted to the hospital with a cancer diagnosis that could be terminal. He was given a large room with a built-in banquette with cushions by a good-sized window. The banquette converted into a bed, and that was where I would sleep that night while my otherwise healthy David occupied the hospital bed. Two friends fetched River, who, by then, had been sitting in the car for hours.

The next day, David would undergo a battery of tests to see if, and to what extent, the cancer had spread.

If you know anything about melanoma, you know it isn't one of the "good" cancers. It's the most aggressive and deadliest form of skin cancer. If it *had* spread to other parts of David's body, that would mean David had stage 4 melanoma. Until very recently, that diagnosis meant *get your affairs in order*, particularly when it was found in the brain. I knew more about melanoma than David did because I'd had a handful of skin cancers burned off my face or surgically removed from other parts of my body. Until that day, David had no idea what melanoma was. He thought it sounded like a tropical drink.

For now, we were both so overwhelmed by the news that we talked about *anything* but cancer. My body vibrated with anxiety, but I tried to appear in control, never sharing with David how scared I was. Instead, as a journalist, I resorted to reporter mode: making lists of who to call and what to pick up, gathering information, making a plan. To deflect the panic, we attacked our to-do lists. We got someone to feed and walk River for the next few days. David emailed his boss to say that he was in the hospital for tests and wouldn't be in the next day. He was working for USAID at the time, flying back and forth between DC and Kabul, and was worried about a favor he'd promised a colleague in Afghanistan. He was supposed to pick up a special medication at a pharmacy here and give it to an office colleague who was flying to Kabul the next day. Most people, I imagine, would decide they'd earned a pass on the favor and apologize for not delivering. But David tracked down another work friend, and she agreed to pick up the medicine. Keeping busy was our elixir.

We needed to tell our kids that we weren't coming to LA. David worried about what he would tell Ted, then twenty-seven. He didn't want to frighten his son; he wanted to reassure him that he was going to be all right, but neither of us knew if that was true. His younger son, Billy, then twenty-five, was in South Africa with his girlfriend, Laurence, and couldn't easily be reached. David decided we should wait until we had more information—maybe the picture wouldn't be so grim tomorrow.

He did get in touch with his ex-wife, the boys' mother. She reminded David that all doctors aren't created equal and emailed him a list of the ten best cancer centers in the United States. At the top was nearby Johns Hopkins in Baltimore. On seeing that, David remembered an old Peace Corps buddy named Rebecca who worked for a doctor at Hopkins. While David called her, I made a list of what we needed from home for our unexpected overnight: phone chargers, laptops, toothbrushes, meds, and toiletries.

When I got back from picking up the items from our apartment, I climbed into the narrow hospital bed with David, and we held each other tightly. Without speaking, we were reassuring each other, letting each other know we were going on this frightening journey together. Somehow, we fell asleep, though I needed help from Ambien, which I would continue to need in the months to come.

We woke the next morning to the standard hospital bustle. Nurses carrying breakfast trays and checking vital signs. Machines beeping. Doctors whose names we didn't catch filing in and out. A constant hectic interruption that kept us preoccupied. Eventually, David was whisked off for scans. While I waited for him to return, I did what I do best: get information. I visited cancer and melanoma research sites and found a blog by a melanoma survivor who lived near us. His name was Wayne Connors, and he ran a support group near us in Alexandria. I emailed him immediately.

I can hardly breathe, I wrote. *We don't have a diagnosis beyond it's metastasized in his brain. We live in Arlington. I saw your blog post. Could you talk with us? Please.*

Four hours later, Wayne emailed us:

Don't get caught up in the median life-expectancy statistics and things like that. They are very scary, and they ARE NOT ABOUT YOU. Every case and every person is different, and for a patient I don't think it does any good to dwell on those kinds of stats…. It's a strange thing to say, but if you have to have melanoma, this is kind of the best time to have it. All these new therapies are changing the treatment of melanoma and having an incredible impact. The last eight to ten years have seen huge advances.

Wayne's advice was sage, and I felt briefly hopeful. But the optimism didn't last. Sometime after David returned from his tests, a doctor came in and said, quite matter-of-factly, that a full-body scan had found sixteen tumors in David's lungs and that it looked like there were spots on his gallbladder. The melanoma that had metastasized to his brain had also spread to other organs. Just like that we'd jumped from stage 2 to stage 4 (there is no stage 5). David had zero symptoms other than the lump on his head. In fact, the previous weekend we'd biked fifty miles. Even in a hospital gown, he was the picture of health.

What we wanted was a plan, someone to fix David's problem, to offer us some hope. We weren't getting clarity at this hospital. David's original melanoma oncologist wanted to start David right away on a clinical immunotherapy trial involving a combination of two new drugs—Yervoy and Opdivo—that the FDA had only approved in 2015. However, it was not known if these drugs could cross the blood-brain barrier. The early results, he said, were promising, so far, showing a synergistic effect that destroyed melanoma tumors in the brain. But the surgeon assigned to us thought we needed to first surgically remove two tumors on one side of David's brain. He didn't have the skill to do both sides of the brain at one time and was offering to remove the two on one side to relieve the pressure. The two doctors' conflicting recommendations made us desperate for another opinion.

In the meantime, David's Peace Corps friend, Rebecca, had already gotten us an appointment for the next day with one of Hopkins' top melanoma specialists. I took on the job of hunting down copies of David's scans to upload into the Hopkins system. I ping-ponged from one unhelpful person to the next until, near tears, I found an IT guy tucked away in a room filled with wires and computer equipment. He was able to help, which he did, generously; it was all I could do to keep from hugging and kissing him. We got the films uploaded and sent to Hopkins. Looking at them, finally, I could see that the cancer was ravaging David's body.

We left the hospital early Thursday morning, having refused both treatments the doctors had suggested. We were giddy as we drove away. It felt like we were breaking out of jail. The Hopkins expert would save us! But in my notebook I wrote, *I am numb/terrified already imagining that I can't/don't want to live without David. Things look bleak.*

2

I Don't Have a Little White Dog

"You have to go on Match.com," my girlfriends insisted. "You've been divorced for a long time. Do you want to spend the rest of your life alone?"

Well, no. But internet dating terrified me. I'd been with my former husband for almost two decades. I wasn't interested in meeting strangers through a screen. I'd already tried the obvious things: I'd joined a weekend biking group, hoping I'd meet someone with similar interests. I'd gone on a few blind dates friends had set up. But—eww. One had been divorced three times and tried to kiss me on the first date. None of them went very far, but they made me anxious.

For someone who likes to think of herself as adventurous, dating brought out the scaredy-cat in me.

Finally, in 2011, I decided to be true to my adventurous side and give it a try. I didn't get more than a few bites, which I found distressing, given that I was in good shape, had a successful career, lots of friends, and owned my own house. I reached out to one potential "match" because I thought we had similar interests.

He responded quickly with, "I don't think we are a match." Really, no one but a guy who owned a coffee plantation in Brazil appeared curious.

"I like to kiss," he wrote.

Me too. But I wasn't going around telling everyone….

I put my weak dating efforts to bed. I wasn't ready. I was happy with my life, friends, family, and my dog, whom I considered great company.

Something shifted, though, during Christmas that year. My niece, Lydia, who I love like a daughter, had gotten married that September. Cutter and I had flown out to Lake Tahoe for Christmas to be with my sister Judy, Lydia's mother. Cutter, Judy, and I were in one house; Lydia was with her husband's family in another. Judy was a single mom and for years had had her three kids to herself on holidays. But one by one they'd married, and I could see how hard it was for her that Christmas morning, with Lydia in the other house, opening gifts with her husband's family.

At the time, Cutter, my only child, was twenty-five. His father and I had long been separated, and he spent most holidays with me. But watching my sister, I looked ahead and saw my future: Cutter would find someone, and he'd spend half the holidays with her family, and I'd be on my own. It sounds melodramatic, maybe, but it made me realize I didn't want to spend the rest of my life alone.

Given the poor response to my first attempt at internet dating, I shared my profile with a good friend who was a Match.com wiz. She'd had dozens of dates and had found a love through the cybersphere. I sent her the profile I'd written under the nom de plume of Writer/Rider, which I thought was very clever given that I was a writer and an avid cyclist.

"This is terrible," she said. "You sound like you don't need anyone. You need to be flirtier and fun."

"How do I do that?" I said.

"Get a white dog," she said, showing me all the pictures of women older than the age of fifty that had white dogs in their photographs.

I didn't have a white dog. River was a black dog, and he was perfect.

She asked me what I was so afraid of, and I told her that I didn't know if I could be flirty and fun, honestly. My last marriage had ended when I came downstairs for breakfast and my then-husband told me that a moving truck was coming for his things at 11:00 a.m. I was blindsided.

By now I had recovered, but the part of me that remembered that moment wasn't sure if I wanted to begin again. I needed to acknowledge that I hadn't been on the dating scene for quite a while and was unsure about how it would go.

"Get over it," she said, not unkindly, and suggested I read a book titled, unforgettably, *Getting Naked Again: Dating, Romance, Sex, and Love When You've Been Divorced, Widowed, Dumped, or Distracted!*

I read the book, which was useful, although the getting naked part did scare me. I no longer had the body of a twenty-eight-year-old, wasn't sure I wanted to open my whole life and family to strangers, and I did worry about my fat bottom.

Still, I gave it another go and wrote a new profile: *I don't have a little white dog*, I began. *I have a big black dog named River. But River can't ride a bike. He doesn't like going to the movies, reading books, or talking about politics. About all he'll do is go for a hike with me.*

In some ways, I knew what I wanted. Someone tall and athletic and who was either younger than I was or no more than two years older. Anyone older than sixty would soon enough require caretaking I figured, and I didn't want to be someone's nurse-with-a-purse. I was adamant about the age limit, which I thought would protect me from becoming a caretaker; it was an irony that would come back to haunt me many times.

David responded to my Match.com profile in January 2012, certain, he later told me, that he'd found a match. He'd been looking for a partner who liked biking and camping, was bright and funny, had a different career than his, and was of a similar age. He, too, loved to cycle long distances. But what endeared me was how he wrote about his two sons, Ted and Billy, both still in college. He adored and was so proud of each of them. It reminded me of how much I adored my son and niece and their friends. I liked that he understood how important children are. And he seemed like someone who enjoyed trying new things.

Still, I wasn't ready to meet him in person. I insisted we email back and forth for a while, gradually getting to know each other through writing. I had emphasized in my profile that I wanted friendship first, and emailing struck me as a safe way to do that. David agreed.

During this period, he went on dates with other women but continued to feel that his No. 1 match was still this woman he'd never met or even spoken to on the phone—me.

For a few months, we shared the details of our lives. His son Ted was in a film program at Emerson College in Boston, coincidentally, the same program my own son had attended a few years earlier. Cutter had dropped out, certain that he didn't need film school. He'd learned a lot about filmmaking in high school, where he'd lucked into a very talented film teacher. He'd already made a short film, *Fishing Without Nets*, about Somali fishermen lured into piracy, which had won the Grand Jury Prize at Sundance that year.

To my surprise, David already knew about Cutter's success. He'd read about Cutter's film online. He had also figured out where I lived and biked by my house—unbeknownst to me. This both fed my fears of sharing my personal life with strangers and attracted me to someone willing to invest such effort in getting to know me. We lived just a mile from each other. Still, for various reasons—my insistence on emailing, David's travel to Afghanistan for a month, my trip to Beirut for a news literacy project—we didn't meet in person until April 1.

David invited me to a Moroccan restaurant for dinner. He'd been in Morocco with the Peace Corps for two years when he was in his twenties and still loved the food. I was nervous going to meet him, but I was also feeling so drawn to him through our email exchanges, I expected to feel the sort of attraction that makes you want to leap across the table. But when I saw him, all I could focus on was the gap between his two front teeth! (It's really not that big.) We had a pleasant enough dinner, where we picked up on threads started in our email discussions. I nervously played with my hair, and at the end, he kissed me lightly on the cheek, and we went our separate ways. While I wasn't smitten, he seemed like a nice guy, and he liked to bike. *Why not have him as a friend?* I reasoned. Better anyway because he wasn't even officially divorced.

David left our date a little disappointed. It hadn't felt perfect, but he didn't know whether that was because he had failed to impress me or vice versa. He still remembers being taken aback by my frequent use of the f-word. He wasn't sure if I was acting tough, was uncomfortable, or really was a hard-ass. It's easy for me to see now that all these things were true: I was in defense mode, acting tough, *and* I was uncomfortable. I didn't want to think I needed anyone. But our two months of sharing over email had left him feeling there was more potential to explore than our dinner date had suggested, and he wanted to get to know me better.

The following weekend I invited him on a bike ride with a friend, my wing-woman. Then I invited him to a movie premiere and another. He was growing on me. At the second movie screening, as I leaned forward to watch, I felt his hand on my back. I froze. He quickly withdrew his hand.

We kept seeing each other, and I kept up a wall, physically. One night we went out, and he dropped me off. I was afraid to invite him in because I thought he would want to have sex, and I wasn't ready for that. When I saw him quickly backing away, I thought he was angry about not being asked to come inside. (I later learned he was just reversing the route he had taken, not knowing his way around.) Finally, after a few weeks of this, he came back to my house because he wanted to go on a walk with River; he said he missed having a dog. The three of us walked through the Columbia Gardens Cemetery a block from my house. Midway through my usual loop, David stopped and kissed me. This time, I surrendered. As I said, it had been more than a decade. The kiss reminded me of everything I'd forgotten I wanted. I felt my body waking up, remembering what I'd been missing. It felt like coming home. But it also felt almost awkward, like I was a teenager again.

A complicated moment.

Over the next three weeks, our relationship blossomed. But then I panicked. I went dark, much to David's shock. We'd gone from zero to sixty, and suddenly I wasn't answering his emails or texts. He didn't know why—because I didn't know why. It just felt like things were happening too fast, and I freaked. Cutter's short film was debuting at a DC theater, and I didn't want David there, which in retrospect feels particularly cruel. Friends and family were coming from out of town, and I thought he wouldn't fit into my life. So just like a millennial, I ghosted him.

By this time, David knew he liked me a lot and had thought it was mutual. We'd enjoyed our time together, and our interests and values seemed very consistent. We laughed a lot. Physically, things were going very well. But maybe, he thought, he'd misjudged the situation. Or maybe I'd just changed my mind. It had been decades since he'd been on the dating market, and he was as confused as I was by my behavior. On the Metro coming home one night, he wrote me a short note:

I have had too much to drink and know better than to write this, but want to tell you how I feel about you. I think you are fantastic. You are smart, pretty, and funny the whole package. What every guy claims they want. You are physical, independent, and open-minded. You are honest, a straight-shooter, and direct. I was worried that you had no softer side, but you finally revealed that to me.... thank you for sharing your life with me.

His note only frightened me more. I didn't respond.

A week later at my book club, somebody asked about my new guy, and I confessed that I had ditched him.

"Why would you do that?" asked my friend, Jenn, the wing-woman who'd biked with David and me and had liked him.

"I'm afraid," I said. "I don't want to get hurt again."

Jenn said that was understandable, but that I should be telling David this, not them.

"Tell him you're scared," she said.

Finally, after the long silence, I texted David. *Can we talk?*

When he agreed, I drove to his apartment. He came downstairs, and we sat outside on the wall. I took a deep breath and started telling the truth. I told him that I had felt abandoned by my father who died when I was eleven. I told him about being blindsided by my ex-husband's departure. I told him that since then I had been on my own for a long time. The idea of having someone care for me and vice versa scared me, and I wasn't sure how to adjust to it. He said he understood. He was scared, too. He hadn't been with anyone but his wife for two decades, and this was all new and frightening to him as well. We talked openly and honestly. By the end of the conversation, we were laughing, hugging, and kissing, closer than we'd ever been, and it felt so liberating.

In an email a few weeks later, I wrote, *I love how honest you are and how you think about things and bring them up later. That's new to me.*

As the months progressed, we fell more deeply in love. We committed to being honest with each other and working to make our relationship succeed. We'd both "bombed" at marriage (David twice!) and swore we'd learn from the communication failures that had led to the demise of those marriages. One thing I loved then—and is something we still often do—was David's insistence that when we talk about something difficult, we hold hands. It's hard to shut down in the middle of an emotionally difficult topic when you're holding hands.

A month later, we were out to dinner and ran into one of my girlfriends, who later texted, *He's hot. You're glowing.* I shared it with David, who asked me what I thought.

I responded, "If my friends repeatedly tell me I'm glowing, then I think you must have something to do with it. They weren't saying that before David Marsden came into my life."

3

Trauma Never Leaves

In the car on the way to Johns Hopkins, I felt a familiar tightness in my gut, the feeling I always got when I was under stress—that feeling that was born not long after my father died. My mother, tough, demanding, and resourceful, who never went anywhere without her "face on" or her unfiltered Chesterfields, quickly moved us to a smaller house and went to work at a series of jobs: demonstrating Mr. Coffee machines at a New Jersey shopping mall, selling real estate, managing an art museum shop.

At that time, I was deeply angry at the world. I was furious at the unfairness of losing my father when so many other fathers were alive and well. I hated the way it seemed as though everyone looked at us with pity. I hid everything—my grief, my fear of losing another person I loved, the way I felt alone—behind a wall of toughness and activity. We stuck out among the families in our world, whose dads commuted from Montclair, New Jersey, to New York City and whose moms were home to greet their kids after school. I blamed my mother. (Why not? Maybe then she'd leave me, too, and I could be right that the world was a shitty place that hurt people.) I was constantly testing her to see if she would leave me. But no matter what I did, she never left me or my brother, for which I love and respect her immensely. She loved me regardless. Something for which I'm still grateful.

Now, racing to another hospital with David, I thought about a time when I was newly married to my first husband and told my mother that I couldn't imagine living without him. She scoffed, took a drag from her Chesterfield, and said, "You'd do what I did. You'd go forward with your life. You wouldn't have a choice."

The Chesterfields ultimately killed her. She died of lung cancer when I was in my forties. I was her caretaker during that terrible last year of her life, through the chemo treatments and radiation, helplessly watching her waste away. She was a piece of work; she could be difficult and needed to be the center of attention, but she was also regal, dramatic, and driven. At sixty-eight, fourteen years before cancer came for her, she decided she wanted to be in soap operas and hit the pavement in New York City. She landed a job as an extra on *One Life to Live*. Later, she got other bit parts and background scenes and acted in commercials. She even appeared in a music video with the rocker Tom Waits. She was a force. I still miss her. Every day. And I couldn't even think about watching someone I loved go through all that a second time.

Yes, I thought now, *I'd go forward with my life.* But I sure as hell didn't want to do it without David. It had been hard enough going forward without her.

David, meanwhile, was checking his phone. He had left messages with both his boys but still wasn't sure what to tell them when they returned his calls. That he had cancer? That he had tumors in his brain and on his lungs and gallbladder? That he was going to be fine? But he was anxious to connect with them, especially Billy, who was overseas.

"I wonder how our kids are doing?" he said.

"Maybe we should schedule a Skype call," I said.

My relationship with David's sons was spotty, awkward, and almost nonexistent. I met Billy early on in our relationship, when we were in Chicago on the way back from a cross-Iowa bike trip. Billy was in the Windy City doing a summer internship, and I insisted that David invite him to dinner so I could meet him. I was so crazy in love with David that I wanted desperately to meet his kids, although now I'm not even sure why it was so critical to me. I pushed and pestered him to include Billy for dinner at a place that served Chicago's famous deep-dish pizza.

David said he wasn't sure the kids were ready for that.

I said, "Come on. I love you. You love me. It will be great. I'll talk sports," I went on, knowing that Billy, like my son Cutter, had a passion for soccer and basketball. "I'll even mention Duke." (His favorite team).

What I didn't really know or understand was that while David's soon-to-be-ex-wife had sanctioned his dating, Billy and Ted had only learned of their parents' split a few months before. David and their mother had lived apart for more than two years while David was in Afghanistan and then working and living in DC. To me, it was clear the marriage had long been over, especially since the two parted amicably and quickly.

But it wasn't as clear to the kids. Billy didn't know all that. He was still processing his parents' split. At dinner, he was guarded, and I talked too much. We were all excruciatingly uncomfortable. Later, Billy told David how angry and hurt he was that his father had forced that dinner on him.

Some months later, Ted indicated he *might* be interested in getting to know me, which was both exciting news and a little intimidating at the same time. I'd heard Ted was wickedly funny, creative, and passionate about filmmaking. I wanted him to like me, but I'd also wanted Billy to like me, and that had been a mess.

I was in Las Vegas at the time, and David flew in from Kabul. I picked him up at the airport, and we drove straight to Los Angeles to meet Ted for dinner. That night flowed more easily than the disastrous pizza night with Billy. We talked about movies, music, and LA life. Beer helped.

Nothing quite gelled, though, and in retrospect, it was all too soon. After those dinners and a failed attempt at getting Ted and Cutter together, David thought it wiser to keep our relationship separate from his with his sons, to give them time.

Once at his apartment during our first year, I overheard him detailing his weekend plans to Billy. My name never came up. It stung, but I got it. As David later admitted, there's no road map for handling divorce, dating, and kids. Even now, years after the Chicago dinner, both David and I harbored an unmet desire for the five of us—us, his two sons, and my son, Cutter—to like each other, be pals, and hang out together. We had settled, unfortunately, for years of polite indifference.

I sat in the car, watching the suburban houses give way to big-box stores as we crossed the state line and moved through Maryland. I wanted to make lists and find solutions and support, the way I always had in the past when things got tough. *Just buckle down, Lisa.* I thought. *Fuck it. You can do this, and you have to.*

David drove along on the beautiful day, commenting on how different this type of travel was from the way we learned to travel in Afghanistan. It was typical David looking at the positive side. And it was also true.

We'd survived living in a war zone. We'd survived tough interactions with each other's children. Maybe just possibly, we'd get through this, but I had no idea how.

4

Afghanistan

Early in 2012, the University of Las Vegas offered me a job as a visiting professor teaching journalism ethics, a subject I'd become an expert in as the National Public Radio's first outside ombudsman (an official appointed to handle outside complaints regarding administration) and as a longtime media writer. I'd accepted the one-year position before I'd even met David, and I certainly wasn't putting that on my Match profile. When I finally confessed that I was moving west for a year that September, his first response was memorable.

"I'm going to keep dating," he said.

But he didn't. We managed to fly back and forth nearly twice a month. When I had my hip replaced at Stanford University in December of that year, he flew there—after spending Christmas with his boys in Cabo San Lucas—to drive me back to Las Vegas. By New Year's Eve, I was certain he'd say the l-word. We'd been together for nine months, and as we watched the fireworks on the Las Vegas Strip from my balcony, I waited hopefully. But it didn't happen. It would take two more months and a bottle of wine before I got up the nerve to tell him that I loved him and ask, "Do you love me?"

In fact, he did. Very much so.

Around that time, David told me that his office wanted him to go back to Kabul and spend a year there. What did I think? Should he take it?

Impulsively, I said, "Yes! I'll find a job there and join you."

My friends and family thought I was crazy. This was 2013. Every few days, headlines blasted the latest Taliban casualties and deadly car bombs. Who *voluntarily* goes to Afghanistan in the middle of an unending, violent war?

Apparently—me.

It wasn't the first time my friends and family thought I was nuts. In 1987, when I was thirty-four, my then-husband Robert and I sold everything we owned, bought a boat, quit our well-paying journalism jobs, and sailed through the South Pacific with our nine-month-old baby.

Robert, forty-two, sailed single-handedly from San Francisco to the Marquesas Islands, on *Yankee Lady*, our thirty-two-foot, cutter-rigged, double-ender sailboat. The Marquesas Islands are the easternmost islands of French Polynesia. He sailed solo for forty days without any communication while Cutter and I waited nervously to hear he'd arrived safely. In July, Cutter and I flew to the Marquesas Islands to rendezvous with Robert. (Yes, our son was named after the kind of boat we owned.)

For three years, we sailed from island to island through the South Pacific to Japan, stopping wherever we wanted, staying as long as we wanted, and meeting amazing local people who welcomed us warmly into their villages. Why? Largely because we were sailing with an adorable baby who learned to walk on a sailboat and captured hearts and smiles wherever we went. We were much less threatening as outsiders traveling with Cutter.

"You are going to do what with a baby?" was a refrain we often heard when we shared our plans, especially from our mothers, though they eventually got on board and even visited us in the Society Islands.

But things happen to children, no matter how much you prepare. That's kind of how life works. Yes, Cutter got sick. I still recall a piercing

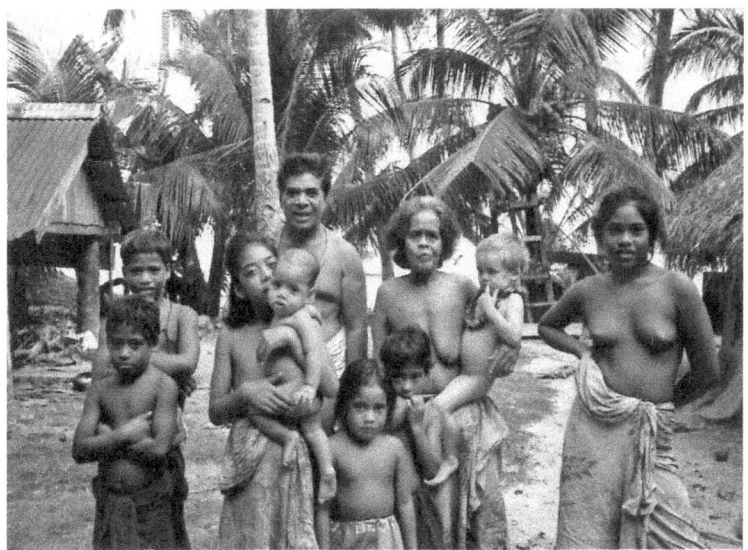

Cutter with a community of friends in the Solomon Islands.

earache on Hiva Oa, an oozing skin infection in Papua New Guinea that rendered him temporarily unlovable, and more than a few bouts with diarrhea. But we stocked up on antibiotics ahead of time and always found the medical help we needed. In one case, a mother on Nuku Hiva in the Marquesas Islands spared me a visit to a medical clinic. She taught me to squeeze water from partially cooked rice that I then fed Cutter in a bottle. The diarrhea cleared up overnight.

Thankfully, Cutter never got sick at sea, though, and I imagine that would have been incredibly frightening. If there were any downside to Cutter's travels, it was that by the time we got to Japan in 1990, he hadn't been exposed to other kids' germs the way most kids are. When he entered a Japanese nursery school at three, he often caught colds. He even ended up in the hospital for five terrifying days with pneumonia in Kagoshima, Japan, where we lived for two years before returning to the United States in 1993. I still feel that sailing with our son was a good thing. We were with him 24/7 for the first three years of his life, and he was a great passport for us to enter local culture.

We both would have done the trip again in a heartbeat and were convinced, despite obvious dangers, that it shaped our boy's thirst for adventure, his willingness to take calculated risks, and most importantly, his curiosity. That said, while my marriage easily withstood and thrived during three years at sea, it couldn't survive suburbia.

Now, in 2014, I was ready for another life-changing journey. And if David wasn't afraid, why should I be? By then, he'd been living amid the Afghanistan chaos for five years and never hesitated to go back—even as it became riskier and there were fewer opportunities to venture outside of the U.S. Embassy fortress compound. He loved the adventure. He loved going back year after year, staying involved with the programs he'd helped initiate and seeing them evolve.

"It's a beautiful country," he said. "You'll love it. The people are friendly, open, and helpful to strangers." He had a lot of respect for them; they'd been through so much and still had high aspirations for their future. It was magical to watch and be a part of.

David's love for working overseas dated back to 1975, when he joined the Peace Corps and went to Morocco. He was working at a dull job in San Francisco and taking business courses at night. He saw where his life was going and didn't like the looks of it, and one night, he expressed his frustration to a friend who told him about the Peace Corps and suggested he apply. The idea totally energized David, who came from a family of travelers. His older sister, Sharon, had quit her job and taken off on a trip around the world with a friend when she was in her twenties. At their mother's request, she bought the younger kids a doll representing each country she visited. They grew up seeing those dolls and being able to name the country they were from. His younger brother, Phil, spent a semester in Asia while at Dartmouth, and then later traveled overland from Thailand to Morocco. The idea of learning a new language and getting to know people from another culture had always appealed to him.

So in summer 1975, he flew across an ocean to a country where he didn't speak Arabic, French, or Berber, nor did he know the customs. After a summer-long language and teacher training in Rabat, the capital, it was time for his assignment. David and a colleague requested a remote post in southern Morocco, near the Sahara Desert and the border of the then Spanish Sahara. They took an overnight bus and arrived at 5:00 a.m. in Tiznit, a village founded in 1881 by the Sultan Hassan. The bus dumped them and their bags (two each) at the town square. No one met them. They were on their own to find a hotel. Eventually, they found a room with only one bed, so David slept on the floor. When they complained about the mosquitoes buzzing around them, a clerk saturated their room with a toxic herbicide. They were too tired to care.

Three days later, David was alone in the tiny village. His Peace Corps mate had slipped on soapy water while washing his hair and cracked his spine. It was up to David, in limited Arabic, to get Paul, who was screaming in pain, help and back to Rabat. Paul was medically evacuated to the United States and never returned to Tiznit.

David spent the next year teaching English to high school classes of twenty-five to thirty students. To help keep his pupils (and himself) engaged, he occasionally used American rock "n" roll songs as teaching tools. Jimi Hendrix's version of "All Along the Watchtower" was a favorite, because to him, it reflected the feeling of being in the village. He would teach his students the English words, and then when everyone had learned what they meant, they'd get to listen to the song. His conversational Arabic dramatically improved, and he became lifelong friends with the principal of the school.

Years later, we visited Morocco and arrived unannounced in Tiznit, at the principal's home. He answered the door and, with as much surprise as pleasure, barked, "Marsden!" Then he engulfed David in a warm embrace, welcoming both of us into his home. They instantly began yakking in Arabic, as if no time had passed, with me interrupting, "What? What is he saying?"

Over the next two days, he took us to his farm, the beach, and restaurants to show how Tiznit had changed in the forty years since David had been there.

As the threat of war with Algeria over the Spanish Sahara increased, David was transferred to Marrakesh for a new assignment as the director of a home and school for children with physical disabilities. For the next year, he worked closely with staff and children, most of whom were orphans and had no other place to live. They had different diseases, but many could not walk without assistance. Most of them lived at the school, which was organized so they had classroom time, physical therapy, and handicraft work, instituted so they could find ways to make a living. David's day-to-day work was ferrying children to doctors, shopping for food and materials for the handicraft workshop, and helping the teachers in the classes. He and John, his fellow Peace Corps colleague, also connected with donors, traveling to Casablanca and going door-to-door to businesses to raise money to run the facility.

To this day, it remains one of the best jobs he says he's ever had.

David would spend a total of six years with the Peace Corps, working four years as a staffer, including three years in Fiji, a stint in the DC office, and his two years volunteering. By the time he was done, he felt like you could drop him anywhere in the world and he would survive.

Business school beckoned, as David learned that although he loved the Peace Corps, he wanted a different challenge than a career in the US government. In 1981, he began an MBA at the University of Chicago with the idea he'd go into international business. But love derailed his international plans, and he got married and remained stateside for the next few decades. After business school, he took a job with Clorox's brand manager training program in the San Francisco Bay Area and eventually held a series of jobs in corporate marketing.

For the next fifteen years, David tried different entrepreneurial ventures, learning a tremendous amount about the challenges of starting a new business. He also spent a lot of time with Ted and Billy, helping with sports teams, music lessons, summer camps, and homework. They loved to go camping together, particularly backpacking in the Sierras.

Once the kids left for college, and David was facing an empty nest, the itch to get back overseas reemerged. USAID was hiring, and the combination of his business and Peace Corps experiences helped him secure a job in Afghanistan in 2009 as a foreign service officer working on economic development.

For the next eight years, he worked both from DC and in-country on programs to encourage business and economic development. This included working with Afghan provinces to develop economic growth plans, encouraging foreign investment through conferences, and introducing modern customs methods and developing trade agreements. He even recruited a number of franchises to come and meet with aspiring Afghans to open offices in Kabul. He had learned over the years not to get too focused on grand ideas of saving the world or reconstructing a completely new government. To him, the change he could effect was made on a smaller scale, through the projects he worked on and person by person. He often talked about how he needed to stay focused on the trees he could help rather than the whole forest.

Typical David.

Lisa Goes to Kabul

So now I had to find work in Afghanistan. David coached me, and I got a two-month tryout gig as a communications manager with the Aga Khan Foundation (AKF), a nonprofit based in Kabul. A week before I arrived in Afghanistan in February 2014, the Taliban killed five people in a bomb explosion at a Kabul police station. The month before, twenty-one died in a Taliban attack on a well-known expat restaurant.

Yet I went.

I went because I feared that my life was becoming a blur of years blending into one another. One Thanksgiving was just like the next. I couldn't remember exactly who was at the table or where it was. I was reaching a point where I couldn't remember what I had done the year before or who I had done it with. My life lacked definition. For the three years we sailed the South Pacific, I can still recall where we were each month. I wanted that challenge and daily adventure back in my life again.

My new assistant, Muslim Khuram (my son's age), met me at the downtrodden Kabul airport when I landed. I was nervous about a stranger picking me up and had insisted via email that we use "peanut butter" as our code word. But like so much of my experience in Afghanistan, this didn't start the way I had planned. He simply introduced himself, and I simply trusted he was who he said and followed him to the car. Looking back now, I see how odd I must have seemed to Muslim, but maybe he was used to terrified Americans arriving in Kabul.

Muslim ferried me through drizzle and mud, past one brown decrepit building after another, past an endless maze of unscalable walls topped with concertina wire. We arrived at a drab guesthouse misnamed the Park Palace, where I was going to stay until the foundation found me a more permanent home. Armed men stood at every entrance. Entering the guesthouse required navigating through standard double-barrier walls. Once through the first door, two men with machine guns scanned my passport and searched my luggage before letting me through the second armed entrance.

Finally, in my room, I unpacked my suitcase but kept putting clothes on rather than taking them off. It was cold inside, and there didn't seem to be a heater. I looked around and thought I definitely was not in Kansas anymore.

On my second night, I was sitting on the floor of my freezing room huddled next to a tiny space heater, my feet jammed into thick wool socks. As I pulled the blanket tighter, I kicked myself for not packing a wool hat. I figured with wearing headscarves, a hat would be a waste of space. It was raining. I was alone, feeling a familiar twinge in my back that harbors spasms to come, and asking myself, *What the hell am I doing here?* The only thing that kept me going was knowing that the next day, a Friday—the equivalent of Sunday in the United States—I would see David. I couldn't wait. I imagined meeting his friends and then having a quiet afternoon snuggling in the warmth of his "hooch"—a trailer with a single bed, desk, bureau, and dorm-size fridge. He said it felt like a single dorm room, although it had its own bathroom.

Our rendezvous could not have gone worse.

I arrived at the embassy compound at 7:45 a.m. The AKF insisted that a driver take me everywhere and pick me up. For safety reasons, there are no signs on the embassy compound, and many guards are Afghan and speak little English. When I asked for USAID, only one of several US agencies in the vast embassy compound, no one knew what I was talking about. I had unwittingly walked way beyond the embassy and gone to the final security check and waited there. No David. Turns out I was at the NATO base.

By the time we found one another, I had been patted down twice by two women. Each time I was stuffed inside a booth the size of a toilet stall and then moved through myriad checkpoints, repeatedly showing my passport.

I was cold, wet, and my back hurt. Instead of falling into his arms with passion, I fell into his bed with a full-on muscle spasm. David had fun plans to show me the grounds, but I slept alone, drugged, until 2:00 p.m. on his single bed. In the afternoon, his friend Jim called wanting to meet me. David told him we were napping. I'm sure Jim thought that was a euphemism. It was not.

At 7:00 in the evening, I finally forced myself out of bed to go see a movie with David. I felt terribly about how the day had gone. David was wonderfully nice and attentive, but I know he was deeply disappointed, too, and frustrated that he couldn't help me. It was the antithesis of the reunion we imagined.

By the time I left at 11:00 p.m., I was still in pain but had run out of pain pills. Nothing was easy in Kabul. There was no doctor for me to call for a refill. Nor was it easy calling for a ride home. I had neglected to write down my driver's dispatch number. It was in my phone. Embassy guards confiscated phones while someone was on US government property. I emailed three colleagues, but while waiting to hear back, the internet went down.

In pain, not knowing my driver's number, I left the embassy, passing through three checkpoints. I walked along a desolate, poorly lit sidewalk the length of a city block to where my driver should have been waiting. When a car arrived, I asked to see the driver's ID to make sure I was getting into the right car, one of many security precautions to which one quickly adapts. As we drove back to my new home, I realized that in spite of everything I felt excited, happy to be there, and very alive.

As bumpy as my introduction to Afghanistan was, David was right. It was beautiful. The weather was almost always sunny, the people were fantastic, the landscape incredible. Behind closed doors, there were close-knit families, amazing craftsmanship, and years and years of people surviving despite the odds against them.

It wasn't the easiest place to have a love affair, and in some ways it was like being in high school. No public display of affection (PDA). Curfews. Check-ins and security ruled our lives.

One evening in late March, an hour before I planned to leave the embassy where I was visiting David, the AKF's security chief, Nasim, called. He said that there was a credible threat planned that night at the Park Palace, where I was living.

"Can you stay at the embassy for the evening?" he wanted to know.

Stunned, I said I'd check and call him back.

David stood there shaking his head. "It's not possible for you to stay," he said.

"Are you kidding me?" I said. "The Taliban plans to attack the building where I'm staying!"

He tried. He called the head of the embassy's vast security team, who said that the best they could do was let me stay until 2:00 a.m.

"Great," I said sarcastically. "Everyone knows the Taliban goes to bed at 1:00 a.m., so that should be fine." I was starting to panic.

David said there was nothing we could do. This was part of living in Afghanistan. If we defied protocol, he could lose his job. The embassy was strictly run, and if any of the set-in-stone rules were broken, one found themselves on an airplane out the next day. A contractor who was found drunk and half-naked in a residence hall was packed up and put on a helicopter to the airport within hours.

I started calling everyone—colleagues, friends, anyone I could think of—to find a solution. Luckily my nonprofit found a safe place for me to spend the night with an American colleague who lived near the embassy. This ended the tension between David and me for the time being, and I kissed him goodbye.

I left, however, feeling angry and confused. I knew the rules needed to be followed, but if David put his job at the embassy over my safety, how was he going to take care of me as we grew old together? And how did I not know he was such a rule follower? I never met a rule I didn't want to break, and this seemed like an especially good time to let protocol go. I was pissed and scared and wondered why I'd even bothered to come.

David was also upset. He felt caught in an impossible situation. He was well aware of the rules and the consequences for disobeying them. He was also acutely aware of the danger I was facing and hated feeling helpless about keeping me safe. He was also slightly annoyed that my security guy even asked. Anyone who'd been working in Kabul for any length of time knew the embassy was not a safe harbor for nonemployees. At the same time, he was proud of me for finding my own solution.

After I texted him about my safe arrival at a friend's house, he felt like we'd passed a major test.

I did, too, and it was the beginning of understanding the extent to which I was going to have to learn to adapt. A few days later, I got a Valentine card from David that buoyed my spirits, reinforcing I was doing the right thing for us.

I don't often say it, he wrote, *but I think about you every day. You came into my life and changed it for the better—so much better. I just love spending time with you—almost doesn't matter what we do. You always say you feel so lucky, but I feel it is me who is lucky. There is a color and texture to my day that wasn't there before you. And I feel so amazingly comfortable with you. I don't forget what you look like when you aren't around (as you sometimes say about me), but I sometimes wonder if we are a dream. I am so grateful for your understanding and patience with my family situation. And you are both willing and excited to join me on this Afghan adventure. Can't wait to share this chapter of life together. So, without further ado, let me say simply that I love you.*

Park Palace was never attacked. The next day, however, I moved to a poppy palace—an ornate, well-protected guesthouse with ten bedrooms, a huge dining hall, and an opulent living area. This and buildings like it were built with poppy money, hence the name. Some of the lights worked. Sometimes the internet worked. I had my own bathroom, which I quickly learned was a luxury.

My daily routine went something like this: A driver would pick me up at 7:30 to take me to work. I'd grab a cup of instant (yes—ugh!) coffee, don a headscarf, and ride ten minutes to the office, go through security to get in, and stay in the building. For lunch we could order in food from preapproved places. (I couldn't leave the premises to go get real coffee or go out and grab something.) The Afghan staff ate food at the office, which I could have done, but it was always the same: rice, meat, and salad.

Around 5:00 p.m., I'd climb into a van with six Afghan staff (there was no public transport in Kabul), and on their way home, I'd get dropped off at the embassy. Traffic was usually bumper-to-bumper in that city of six million. There were no traffic lights. The main roads were okay, but the side roads were muddy ruts that required four-wheel drive and holding on. We'd pass by a combination of residential, commercial, and industrial buildings, all interconnected, and each a mix between old, new, and ancient—the history of the dramatic changes the city had undergone visible in a single commute across town.

At the embassy, I'd go through three checkpoints: the first two with Afghan guards who spoke little English, the last with embassy personnel. I'd get a red V (for visitor) badge, David would come to get me, and then we were on the property. Together. But no kiss hello. No hug. No PDA. He had to accompany me everywhere, which I might have minded in the United States, but here, where I didn't know my way around or know the customs, I enjoyed it. Knowing this unique experience was something David and I would share forever made it even richer.

Most days we worked out in a fabulous gym and ate in one of three dining facilities. Brunch on Fridays was something to look forward to: fresh homemade cinnamon rolls, chocolate milkshakes, bacon, and omelets made-to-order sitting by the Olympic-size swimming pool. For me, there was a mental disconnect, seeing the bronzed, muscular bodies of security personnel frolicking in the pool, drinking and tanning in skimpy suits, as we ate delicious American food poolside. It seemed like spring break; when outside it was all drab—headscarves and burkas.

Some days I'd go back to my guesthouse, walking through streets with literally no name, looking out for packs of wild dogs that roamed the city like they owned it, and I'd think people at the embassy, while well-intentioned, had no idea what it was like for their Afghan colleagues. (On the other hand, I often saw armed and vested security/military personnel preparing to go out somewhere, and I was awed by their courage as they prepared to leave the compound.) Often David introduced me to his friends by saying, "This is Lisa. She lives in the real Kabul. You don't really live in Afghanistan on the embassy."

I worked for the AKF for three months, and then got a job at Impassion Media, a digital news group developing citizen journalists. It was started by smart, young Afghans educated abroad. Their hip, modern offices and expensive, tailored clothes put into stark relief how Stone Age the rest of Kabul felt at times, with unpaved roads, men in turbans, women's heads covered, some in floor-length blue burkas. Donkeys pulling carts down the street. One of the partners was a young woman, an American—brave, entrepreneurial—who zipped around the streets of Kabul on a motorcycle. *These guys are the future,* I thought.

I moved out of my poppy palace and into a simple residential house with a lovely garden, with two other people from my office, both about my son's age. What was cool to me was that we hung out together, regardless of the age difference, drinking, dancing, having fun. It was just life in Kabul where we "One-Offs" (the name given to people who come for a one-year term and then leave, which was most Westerners) lived. The place was full of characters—weirdos searching for adventure, me included.

Over the next year, I worked as a writer, an editor, and an election observer; experienced lockdowns many times; and got to explore a stunning country that would have terrified me had I only seen it through the lens of the nightly news.

Once, for work at the AKF, we had to film a video for a Japanese donor. We drove to the Wakhan Valley, surrounded by Pakistan to the south, Tajikistan to the north, and China to the east. Goats, cattle, and donkeys occasionally blocked our path. What stood out to me were farmers in the field turning the soil with two yaks and a wooden tiller. Our driver dropped us off near the border with Tajikistan, and we walked with luggage and equipment to the other side, going through customs. No metal detectors. Very low-key. The guards asked us to stay for tea.

Later, I met a smart young man who had gotten into Kabul University eight years previously. To get to the town where he could board a bus, he had to walk with his family for three days.

Often, Afghans would see my iPhone and demand I snap them. They never smiled. Very proud.

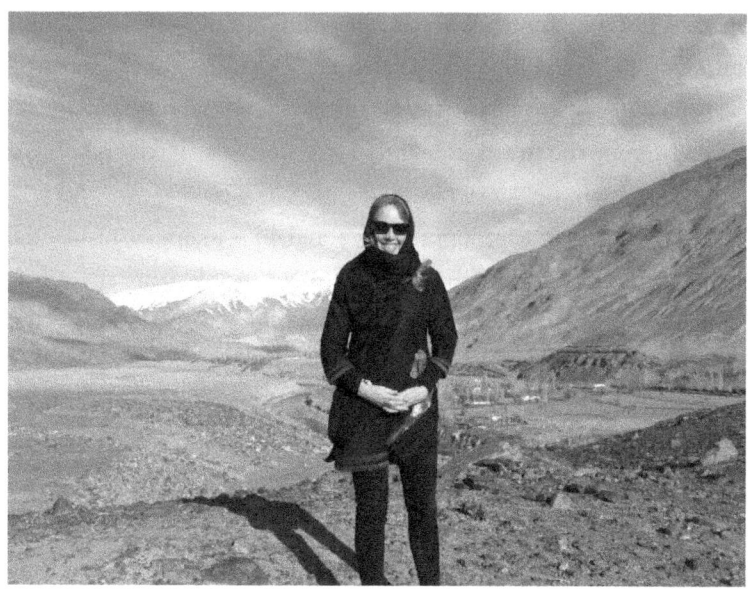

Me with my film crew in the Wakhan Valley in Afghanistan.

Another time, my colleague Noori, twenty-six, invited me to celebrate Eid al-Fitr—a major three-day holiday that marked the end of Ramadan—with his family. It was like a combo of Thanksgiving and Christmas: gifts for children, visiting family, eating and eating and eating.

Noori picked me up with his two young nephews, and we drove twenty minutes to where his family had owned property they could trace back six hundred years. (Yes, six hundred!) I wanted to bring my roommate Nick, but a traditional Muslim woman could not be in the same room with a man who was not her relative, so Nick's presence would have meant the family could not eat together.

At Noori's family's house, we had tea, mangoes, and grapes. Peaches from their trees. We piled into a car with his three sisters all dressed in Afghan finery to visit another sister. More tea. Fanta. Fresh Afghan melon, mangoes, cake, and cookies. Then off to sister No. 5, who was about to deliver a baby. More cookies and cakes and fruit. Always sitting on floor cushions. Much staring, trying to communicate, laughing. (Only Noori could really understand English.) We visited in the overdecorated pink bedrooms of each sister and her husband.

Ten hours later—after going through nine checkpoints because attacks were more likely during Eid when crowds were together—I was home, exhausted, and thankful for the experience.

I was thankful for all of it. Afghanistan was nothing like I thought it would be, but in so many ways, it was more than I ever hoped. I knew it would be an adventure, I knew it would be complicated, I knew it would be dangerous and frustrating. And it was all those things. It was also beautiful, exciting, inspiring, and heartbreaking. Terrible things happened all the time. People got killed. After a while, you got inured—*only six people killed in that explosion,* or *at least they were shot, not tortured.* One woman I wrote a story about went to work one day and, when she got home, found that the Taliban had killed her husband and teenage sons. I am still sick over that.

And yet I was drawn to it. Because as anyone who has ever lived there will tell you, there's just something special about Afghanistan. I don't know exactly what it is—the ancient mountains with their breathtaking beauty or how warm and strong the people are, especially the younger generation, who exude entrepreneurial enthusiasm and grit. Or the way modernity and antiquity live side by side. Or all of it.

I do know that if you go to Afghanistan, you will be astounded by the vibrant energy thriving in that country that will not give in to war.

In November, I got yet another job training journalists. I was sad to leave my digital start-up and team of twentysomething Afghans. On one of my last nights, we launched a website I'd helped create that would track the first one hundred days of President Ghani's administration. I stayed at the office till 12:30 a.m., powering through the glitches, eating pizza, and drinking Coke and getting it done in the midst of a three-hour power outage.

It was everything I loved about journalism—working with a team of smart, young people, writing about significant events. To my surprise, I was having the time of my life.

A week or so later, I hosted Thanksgiving at the guesthouse. I invited all of my Afghan friends and colleagues and wrote about it in a series of letters I'd sent back home called "Dispatches from the Love Front."

I'm excerpting it here—slightly edited for brevity.

Saturday, Nov. 15, 2014

Had Thanksgiving with the Impassion staff (the digital media company) and a kind of going-away party for me... I really love this team... Impassion owner, an American, brought back two bags Pepperidge Farm stuffing and Bisquick at my request. Made a huge batch of my mom's stuffing along with cinnamon rolls... Did I mention the propane stove has only high and low? So no idea what the temperature was. Threw (a turkey) in at 1:30. Everyone to arrive at 3:00 p.m. My fear was not enough meat on the bird for twenty people... same pre-party panic I have in United States: There won't be enough food.

I knew that whatever happened, it would be fun. And it was. Staff loved the turkey... The folks who work at Impassion Afghanistan... are my kind of people. Hardworking, lots of joking and laughs and great attitudes. Miss them.

I really do love living here—even with the occasional bomb blasts, limited social world, and security restrictions.... So many Afghans I've met are truly funny. I admire their stamina and perseverance. They all have harrowing tales of living here. When there's a suicide bomber, their families call, equally worried as you all are (about me). This is their home. I can leave; they can't.

What I can't really comprehend is what it would be like to live in a country where you can't leave Kabul to go visit your village because the Taliban are there. Imagine you grew up in New Jersey, but live in Connecticut, and could never go back to where you grew up because you might be killed. (No NJ jokes, pls.).... Every day is an adventure.... My commute is about thirty minutes, so I find myself mesmerized by all the sites as I drive by.... It seems fine to not be able to get out and walk around. That doesn't bother me.

So our multicultural Thanksgiving dinner was a success. I asked everyone to say what they were thankful for: many said for the peaceful transition to a new government. One for his new son. I continue to pray for a greater sense of security for the folks here. I hope one day, they will no longer worry....

Gobble Gobble,
Lisa

After everyone went home, I sat in the garden. I knew this was one Thanksgiving that would not blend in with the others. I knew I would remember exactly where we were and who was there. (I still do.) My life had more definition. I had daily challenges, adventure, and love. I would always be grateful to David for bringing me there.

And I was grateful, also, to Afghans for teaching me this: In a country like Afghanistan, you have to develop a Zen attitude. When there is no plan, have a plan A, B, or C, or at times, let the plan form on its own. Nothing was easy; everything was a challenge. *I have US dollars. How will I get Afghanis (their money)? I want mangoes, but I can't just walk out on the street to buy them. But I can give a guard money and send him, or ask an Afghan friend for fruit.*

I liked figuring it all out and finding new ways to survive and be happy. I took nothing for granted. I was very careful. All expats were, as were the security people hired to protect us. What we couldn't control was the random event. But you never can, and this would come back into my awareness again and again as time went on.

5

A Constellation of Strangers

As we pulled into the parking lot at Johns Hopkins, David's cell phone rang. It was Dr. Michael Lim, a Hopkins neurosurgeon, calling from Korea. He had David's scans.

"I can't see these in detail," he said, "but I'll be back in the States tomorrow and can talk to you about them then. I think I can help you."

We got out of the car with a spring in our steps. Just the words, "I think I can help you," were all it took to energize us as we walked in to meet with the oncologist.

In the hospital, we met with Dr. William Sharfman, who helped create the Melanoma Program at Hopkins in 1994. We hoped he would be able to treat David with a single surgery followed by immunotherapy. It's often difficult for cancer-fighting drugs, mainly chemotherapy, to penetrate what's known as the blood-brain barrier and get into the brain. Immunotherapy drugs release the brakes on our immune cells that prevent them from attacking cancerous tumors. Early results were promising for a synergistic effect that destroyed melanoma tumors in the brain, or at least that's what the doctor at the first hospital had told us.

But Sharfman was hesitant. Immunotherapy would cause swelling in David's brain and with six tumors, there might not be enough room for the swelling. Brain swelling—or cerebral edema—could cause both long-term and life-threatening effects. Something to avoid.

He spent almost three hours with us, calmly and carefully talking us through options.

I am still grateful to him for this.

The next day, we met Dr. Lim, who we'd spoken with on the phone in the parking lot. He had successfully removed tumors from three sides of the brain at the same time and thought surgery was the best next step for David. Sharfman and Lim sold us on a double craniotomy to fish out the three biggest tumors, followed by a Hopkins trial using targeted radiation and one immunotherapy drug, Opdivo, which received FDA approval for advanced melanoma in 2014.

I still wasn't sure about surgery. "What about the side effects?" I said.

Dr. Lim was blunt. "David *may* die in surgery," he said. "But he *certainly* will die if he does nothing."

We agreed to surgery the following Monday, on March 6, 2017.

We now had a plan but were still in shock. *It's okay*, I kept telling myself. *I can do this. I'll take off work. I'll commute back and forth.*

But who was going to take care of River? Would David need at-home health care after the surgery? Could I even do this, with no help?

David was quiet, so I could see that he was worried, too.

The phone rang. It was Billy, calling from South Africa. He and Laurence were at the airport and would be in Arlington the next day.

An hour or so later, we found out that Ted and Cutter were coming, too.

Without our asking, each son insisted on being there for the surgery.

Others were coming to help, too. David's brother, Phil, was coming up from Atlanta. His friend Rebecca offered to let us all stay at her house nearby while David was going through treatment.

We both felt humbled, overwhelmed with relief, and supported. I felt like we now had a team coming together to help. These were exactly the people we wanted to be with us and each other—but, of course, not for this reason.

Later, I asked each of the boys and Laurence what they remembered from when they first learned about David's melanoma. Not surprisingly, each experienced it differently, depending on how they were told.

Billy had no idea what melanoma was and, when he started Googling it, concluded that his dad was going to die. He was desperate for more information, to find out what the odds were of David surviving.

He had called his mother, who said wisely, "No one knows the answer to that, Bill. If anyone could tell you, they would."

Laurence did her own research, saw that the situation was urgent, and began making plans to come back from South Africa.

Ted felt whiplashed. He had been expecting both of us in LA that weekend. When we FaceTimed with him at the coffee shop where he was working, he thought he was going to hear us at the airport saying we were on our way. Instead, he saw David in a blue-green hospital gown, smiling, telling him calmly that he had cancer in his lungs and his head. Ted remembered leaning on the wall outside the coffee shop and then sliding to the ground and crying.

Meanwhile, I had called Cutter from the emergency department where David was first diagnosed, and I was crying so hard that he started crying, too. All he kept thinking about was the family and how sad this was for everyone. Every little bit of, *We can fight this,* in his brain was met with, *Bullshit, Dave is going to die very soon, and Mom isn't going to be okay.* He spent the rest of the night in his apartment imagining how lonely Dave must be, facing this tidal wave of fear and uncertainty in his own body.

All of us were scared. All of us were glad to be together. All of us knew one thing: We would do whatever it took to keep David alive.

Over the next few weeks, the five of us—Cutter, Ted, Billy, Laurence, and me—formed an impromptu support team. Billy and Laurence moved into the second bedroom in our apartment in Arlington, Virginia. They provided boatloads of emotional support by shopping and cooking for us, walking River, and coming to every doctor's appointment. As San Francisco consultants, they applied their top-notch analytical skills to intensely researching stage 4 melanoma and asked hard questions. The week before surgery, David prepared his will, power of attorney, and medical directives. We even squeezed in another opinion through a Northwestern University contact from David's nephew, Alex. He agreed that surgery was the right way to go.

Our challenges were only just beginning, but David's attitude was amazing. He had full confidence in his medical team and was certain the surgery would work. The night before his surgery, he sent out this email:

> *T-minus one day: There's an enemy residing within me, aka a terrorist organization that goes by the name Stage Four Melanoma. It's made a threat on my life. It's been operating inside my brain and lungs on a secret mission. But it made a mistake and made itself known. My plan: Total Annihilation. We are going to punch it out like Will Smith punching that alien in Independence Day.*
>
> *—Love, Supreme Commander Dave Marsden*

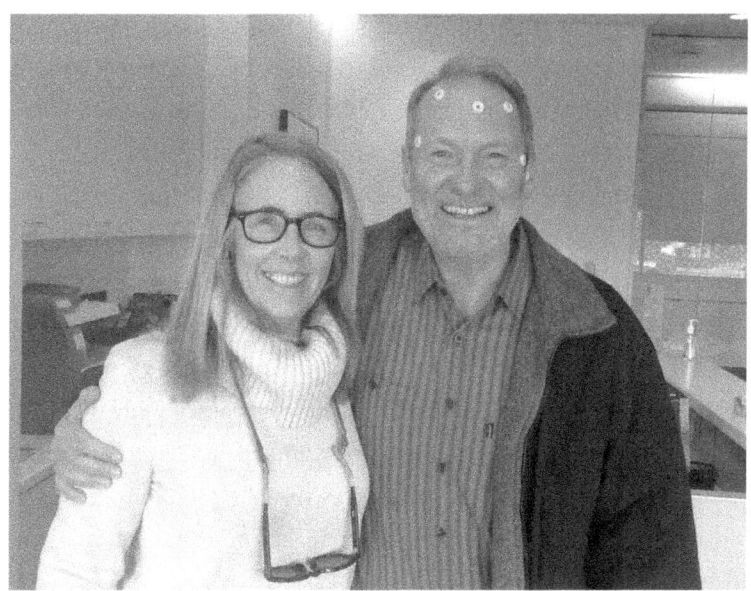

David and I just before surgery on March 6, 2017. The circles are to instruct the neurosurgeon where to set up for the surgery.

Privately, the support team (aka us) was not as assured. The surgery took four, long, stomach-knotting hours. We paced. We walked all over the hospital grounds. We fidgeted. We worried. Finally, Dr. Lim appeared. We huddled around him.

"I got the tumors out," he said, "just in time—not hours, but within weeks of a catastrophe."

A catastrophe? Wow. He explained that the tumors were wrapping around David's blood vessels and risked causing a stroke or seizure.

"When can we see him?" we all said nearly at once. I started crying immediately and was hugged by Cutter, and then everyone—a real group hug of relief. Then people started getting on their phones to let others know.

The recovery wasn't as easy as Dr. Lim had promised. In fact, for a few days, David's condition was terrifying, at least to me.

His brain had swollen, making simple tasks difficult. He couldn't communicate clearly. Each time a doctor or nurse came into the room, they'd ask David a simple question: *What day is it? Do you know where you are?* But he didn't know. He would nod, smile, sometimes say something nonsensical like, "I am here." He couldn't grasp what was happening. Everything confused him. His quick sense of humor had disappeared. It was clear to all of us that the old David wasn't at home.

We used a whiteboard to explain family relationships. David understood better if we drew a family tree or wrote things down. This was especially hard on Phil, his younger brother. Only two years apart, they had always been best friends, and I could see how it pained Phil to see his brother like this. It was troubling to see someone so smart, with a long successful career in business and international development, so confused and lost.

I was struggling, too. The David I knew and had fallen in love with had slipped off to some unrecognizable place. The energy that had ricocheted and pulsed between us as lovers was gone, and I found it so hard to connect with this stranger whose head was wrapped in a turban of white bandages. I would lie down next to him on his hospital bed and whisper in his ear repeatedly, "Come back to me. Please come back to me." He would smile blankly, nodding as though I were a kind lady who had brought him a gift.

He was also uncharacteristically mean and at times rude to the nurses. When Cutter told him he could only have a few drops of water because his sodium level was low, he snapped, "This is bull#@$%! I want water!"

When I tried to encourage David with his walker, he dismissed me like a gnat, telling me to get away. He only wanted his brother.

Was this permanent? We didn't know. No one was telling us anything that I found particularly reassuring. But during those twelve-hour days at the hospital, what gradually changed was the

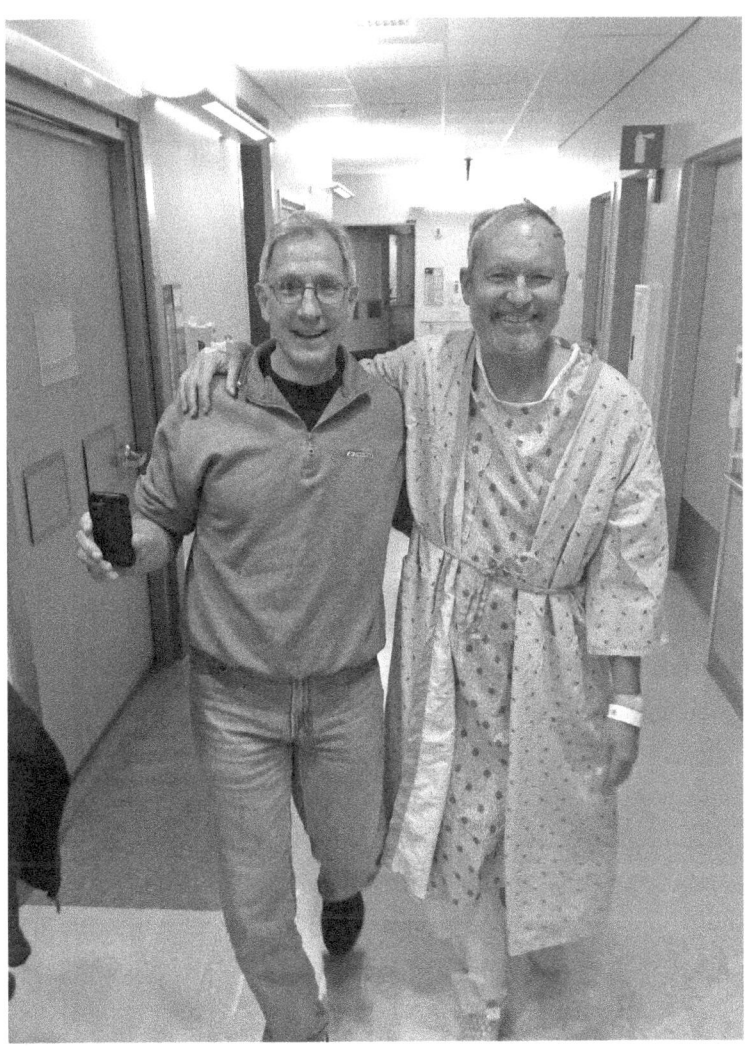

David and his brother, Phil Marsden, postsurgery.

relationships between me and David's kids and the kids with each other. Each day, we'd go off for meals in different configurations, or we'd take breaks and go for walks together when David needed privacy or was taking a nap. We found ourselves, although we never would have wanted it to come about this way, in the situation David and I had always wanted: All of us hanging out. Talking about our lives. Ted was trying to figure out whether to take a job. He sat in the room with David, going over the pros and cons with us. We listened, gave our thoughts. A nurse would walk in and check David's stats, then we'd go back to chatting.

It was strange, Ted said later, that without David being fully present, we got to know each other as people—not as "my dad's new girlfriend" or "my dad's new girlfriend's son."

"I've never heard Dad curse this much," Ted said one day when we were sitting in the café.

"I know," I said. "Who knew that was even in there?"

"At least he's yelling at everyone, so you don't have to take it personally," said Ted. He was referring to Cutter trying to help David get water by giving him a damp sponge on a popsicle stick.

"Welcome to the family," Billy said drily.

"Thanks," Cutter replied.

We leaned on each other like this for days. When I perceived something a doctor said as bad news, Billy and Laurence, in particular, calmly talked me down from the ledge. When Ted worried over breakfast that he couldn't help his dad, Cutter and I pointed out how tender and patient he was with his dad, how much he made him laugh.

Laurence made a spreadsheet of David's medications and prescriptions so everyone could keep track of them. Later, Billy would say that's when he knew he would marry her. If she could show up like that, she was someone he wanted to have by his side forever.

One night, Cutter, Ted, and I returned late to our friend Rebecca's house near Baltimore. She and her husband were generously putting six of us up so we didn't have to go back and forth from Arlington. I was completely drained at that point. Each day in the hospital with David was a little different, but he wasn't coming back to himself as fast as any of us wanted. I got into the door at Rebecca's, and for whatever reason, it all hit me—the fear, how much I hated seeing my partner in pain, how completely exhausted I was. I started sobbing so hard I couldn't stop. Ted, the kid I'd once felt nervous around, sat on my right on the couch. My son sat on my left. They both put their arms around me, hugging me hard. They didn't try to shush me.

"Let it out," Ted said.

I wailed so loudly I woke up our hosts, who got up and poured stiff glasses of bourbon for all of us.

A few days later, I saw a glimpse of David's old self. He was sitting up in his hospital bed watching something on the TV as the nurses came and went.

"When is my brain going to get better?" he asked. "Days? Weeks?"

"Probably weeks," Billy said.

"Weeks? Really?" He paused, thinking. Then he smiled. "Well. #%$@. My brain is pissing me off."

There he is. He's coming back.

A Stroke of Luck

Amid this tense week I emailed Ed, the tenant renting my Arlington house, about why I was late renewing his lease. David would have kept personal details to a minimum, but I am an oversharer by nature and told Ed what we were going through.

He wrote back saying that he represented the Melanoma Research Foundation, a patient advocacy organization that had connections to leading melanoma researchers and research institutions all over the country.

I'm sure you're on top of this, he wrote. *But in case you need a second opinion or referral, I can connect you and David with our network of cancer/melanoma researchers.*

I was overwhelmed by my good luck. I mean, what were the chances? We were woefully uneducated on how to make the *right* decision—a common position for anyone suddenly thrown into a world filled with medical jargon and contradictory recommendations. And here was someone who wasn't a lobbyist for breast cancer, or pancreatic, or prostate—he worked on behalf of getting more funding for melanoma!

That afternoon, from David's hospital room, Billy and I spoke with a doctor at the Melanoma Research Foundation. She recommended getting yet another opinion on David's treatment plan and said Memorial Sloan Kettering and Georgetown's Lombardi Comprehensive Cancer Center were doing cutting-edge work on melanoma with immunotherapy.

Six long, tiring days later, we drove home. In the garage, I couldn't find the keys to our apartment. David glared at me with unfamiliar fury as though I'd sold them for drugs. This time, Billy came to my rescue, putting his arm around me.

"Dad, stop it! You are being a jerk."

Later that night, I reminded David of Billy's kindness. He had no recollection of speaking harshly but recognized his son's protective response was a good thing.

Yet Another Opinion

A few days later, on March 14, 2017, we had a consultation with Dr. Michael Atkins, who had spent more than thirty years ignoring many medical naysayers, steadfastly researching and believing in immunotherapy's promise. Atkins was recruited in 2012 from Harvard Medical School to develop Georgetown's cancer immunotherapy program.

Billy, David, Laurence, and I crowded into his cramped examination room at Georgetown. Since David was asymptomatic, meaning he was healthy and hadn't had a stroke or shown any effects from his brain tumors, Atkins wanted us to join his trial, CheckMate 204. The trial involved thirty-five different medical institutions, all testing whether the two-drug immunotherapy cocktail of Yervoy and Opdivo could shrink tumors in the brain. If we chose to do it, Bristol-Myers Squibb, the drug manufacturer, would cover the costs.

We were hopeful. Billy and Laurence peppered Dr. Atkins with questions evaluating both him and the trial. I just wanted to know if this was a better option for David.

Atkins said that since 2013, about 70 percent of patients who used the double-dose were alive two to three years later, and more than half are likely cured. This sounded great until we learned that there were only about one hundred patients in the study. Not exactly a huge number.

Atkins also said if we did join the trial, David wouldn't need radiation. Three months ago, he explained, he would have recommended it, but protocols were changing rapidly as CheckMate 204 results flooded in.

"One of the things we're really confident about now is *not* doing radiation," he continued.

Though effective, radiation could have long-term side effects such as memory loss, which we all wanted to avoid, if at all possible.

David sat quietly, wearing a black bandanna pirate-style to protect his Frankenstein-stapled, shaved head. He barely asked any questions, likely still unable to absorb the complex medical recommendation. The rest of us bombarded Dr. Atkins with questions.

Now what to do? We still had Hopkins suggesting radiation and an immunotherapy drug, while Georgetown was suggesting we forgo radiation and do a two-drug combo only.

The next day, the four of us trooped back to Hopkins for a meeting with the radiation oncologist, who said there was a slight chance of radiation impacting David's personality and a slight chance of him losing his vision. This scared us. David's brain was already so roughed up from surgery that he required speech and occupational therapy.

During the hour-long drive home, we talked about what to do. Should we go with Hopkins or Georgetown? While Laurence reviewed the research results, Billy talked about the differences between targeted versus whole brain radiation versus no radiation. I sat in the front seat, listening to everyone, trying to hold it together. *Buckle down, Lisa,* I thought. *You can do this. All we need is a plan. All you need is to get through this day.*

When we walked into the apartment, River greeted us excitedly, wagging his tail. Nearby on the floor was an empty wrapper from a one-pound bar of dark chocolate—the equivalent of poison for a dog. I raced him to the vet, unable to hold back my tears.

"The dog ate chocolate and the man I'm in love with has cancer," I said. "I have to decide between radiation treatment and drugs that could save him or might kill him."

The vet was sympathetic, and then turned his focus to the dog. He wanted to give River charcoal to make him vomit.

"Leave him," I was told. "Come back in thirty minutes."

I walked outside and called Cutter, sobbing, gulping air. "David is dying. River is dying," I said. "What did I do wrong? Why is this happening?"

Cutter listened as I cried, and then in a calm, soothing voice, my son became the parent.

"Take a deep breath, Mom," he said. "The two things are not connected. No one is punishing you. River is going to be fine." And River was, $500 later, after spending the night at an animal hospital to be monitored.

Okay, I thought. *We can do this.*

I remembered what Cutter had said. No one was punishing me. All we needed to do was get through each day.

A Decision

When we returned to Georgetown a week later, David's cognitive ability had improved. He was clear on one thing: avoid radiation if at all possible.

Dr. Atkins had us meet a patient who had been in the trial for a year. Her tumors were gone. While most melanomas occur on the skin, it also shows up in eyes, mucous membranes, anus, nails, mouth, or feet. Hers had been discovered from ankle pain.

Talking to another patient who had success from the same treatment made us feel much better about the trial. We then consulted with a Melanoma Research Foundation doctor, who told us to do whatever we were comfortable with. Once we made our decision, he advised, we should embrace it 100 percent.

We landed on Georgetown. It was nearby and convenient. The treatment was free. If it didn't work, we'd return to Hopkins. Most importantly, we had what all advanced cancer patients want: options and hope!

6

Recovery Is a Rough Road

Now that we had a plan, Billy and Laurence decided to return to San Francisco.

We were bereft at their leaving. It had been so comforting having them there every day; I knew I was going to miss them.

I was also scared to be without them and worried that I'd grown too dependent on them. Personality wise, I was not cut out to fight cancer in the same way David, Billy, and Laurence were. They could compartmentalize—break down the steps, strategize, take things one step at a time. In a crisis, they tended to choose controlled calm. I, on the other hand, was a catastrophic thinker.

Anyone in my family will tell you: I generously project dire medical outcomes on friends and family. A persistent headache is a brain tumor. When my sister had a hacking cough that wouldn't quit, I was certain she had lung cancer. (She had tuberculosis.) Generally, I ascribe the worst possible outcome to any symptom.

As Billy once noted, I'm an "impressive worrier."

Beyond that, though, I had been through this once already with my mother. While parts of me knew I could handle it—I could make phone calls, ask questions, do research, and find support—I also knew how draining it was.

All of this might have been okay if David was his old self and we were fighting this together. But he wasn't. Sometimes he was mean, or distant and short, very quick to anger. I often didn't know who I was dealing with. I'd remind him he needed to put on sunscreen and wear a broad hat before we went for a walk. Sometimes he just did it; sometimes he told me to stop trying to control him. I'd see glimpses of him in there, but often he seemed like a stranger. Some days I felt like a servant; getting up to make him salmon eggs for breakfast, cooking special meals for him to adhere to an anticancer diet. He'd be polite and say thank you, but there was no connection. Except in bed, when we snuggled together the way we always had.

Meanwhile, I was constantly worried. What if the immunotherapy didn't work and he died? What if he lived but was never himself again?

It was hard doing all of it alone.

But I was not alone for long. To our surprise, our three sons, along with David's brother Phil, crafted a schedule. Each one would return for a week. Ted came first, cutting short a vacation in Spain. He drove David to and from his appointments for speech and occupational therapy, giving me time to work. I had taken on a huge writing project, which I needed both for the money and for my own sanity. When I could focus, it was a satisfying distraction.

Ted got a front-row seat to see how rough things were when David turned on me one night after I told him not to use Uber.

"Don't tell me what to do!" he yelled, giving me the finger as he slammed the bedroom door.

I burst into tears.

Was it the steroids he was taking to reduce brain swelling, which some people say cause roid rage? Or the aftereffects from the anesthesia? Or the brain surgery? Whatever it was, it wasn't fun.

Ted put his arm around me. "I know this is hard," he said. "We are so lucky to have you taking such good care of Dad. I really appreciate it."

Later, I could tell Ted had said something to his father about being kinder because the next night I found flowers from David.

I appreciate your letting me cry on your shoulder and giving your old man a pep talk, I texted Ted later. *I'm glad you're in my life.*

I really appreciate you taking the time and dedication to take care of my dad, he wrote back. *And I'm glad you're in mine.*

The other challenge was David's ability to communicate clearly. As a result of his surgery, he had something called "anomic aphasia," which is an inability to recall nouns quickly and often confuses them. He could describe someone or a thing in many ways, but it would take quite a while to remember the name.

"A man! A rock and roll singer, very popular, lots of women loved him, lived in Memphis, I even remember how he died," David said one day in speech therapy, trying to say Elvis. "Elvis!" he said, twenty-five minutes later.

"I'm going to Trader Joe's for slim ducks and scotch potatoes," he said another morning as he headed to the grocery store.

Ted looked at me.

"He means salmon and sweet potatoes," I said. (By then I had gotten good at translating for him.)

We played twenty questions or other word games to exercise his brain. One night, we were playing a game where the question was, "What's a new baby called?"

"New, new, new... nuisance!" exclaimed David.

No one could argue with that.

This was my new normal. One day I was crying, the next I was laughing. I was exhausted and trying to be a caretaker and continue working and living a normal life.

One night, Laurence sent me a text asking me how I was doing, and I let everything out.

Not well, I said. I was very anxious. *He's sleeping all the time*, I wrote. *And today has a headache and generally feels lousy.*

It seemed like each day, there was something new to deal with. If it wasn't his head, it was his back. David might seem positive to everyone else, but at home he was depressed, and it was constantly up to me to lift his spirits. I knew I should be more patient, but frankly, it was hard to take care of someone who was mean to me.

She wrote back saying she was sorry to hear that things were hard and reminded me that it wouldn't be like this forever.

You'll both have time to figure out your relationship again in a few months, she wrote. *But it's likely not right now. Which totally sucks for you in that the relationship has now swung to what David needs and not what you need, but in the very long, long-term, hopefully that will right itself. So in the short-term, you need to find support outside of Dave.*

Of course, she was right. I emailed David's Georgetown nurse saying I needed help, hoping Georgetown offered support. She gave me the name of a therapist, but I couldn't get an appointment for weeks, so I gave up. Even when Billy and Laurence gently hinted and pushed me to get support, I didn't.

When you're in that mode of taking care of things, getting help just seems like another in a long line of overwhelming tasks. In retrospect, I did myself, David, and our family a disservice by trying to do it all alone and not taking care of myself. It's a rookie caretaker mistake.

The weekend before David started his immunotherapy treatment in April, we celebrated our fifth anniversary at a Moroccan restaurant. Just us. Giving us a chance to reconnect. We talked about how much we loved each other, how lucky we were, and how compatible. One lovely evening in a sea of angst.

After Ted left, Cutter arrived, hugging me hard.

Finally, on April 4, David got his first dual-drug infusion at Georgetown. Cutter and I watched as the immunotherapy drugs that we hoped would save his life dripped into David's arm.

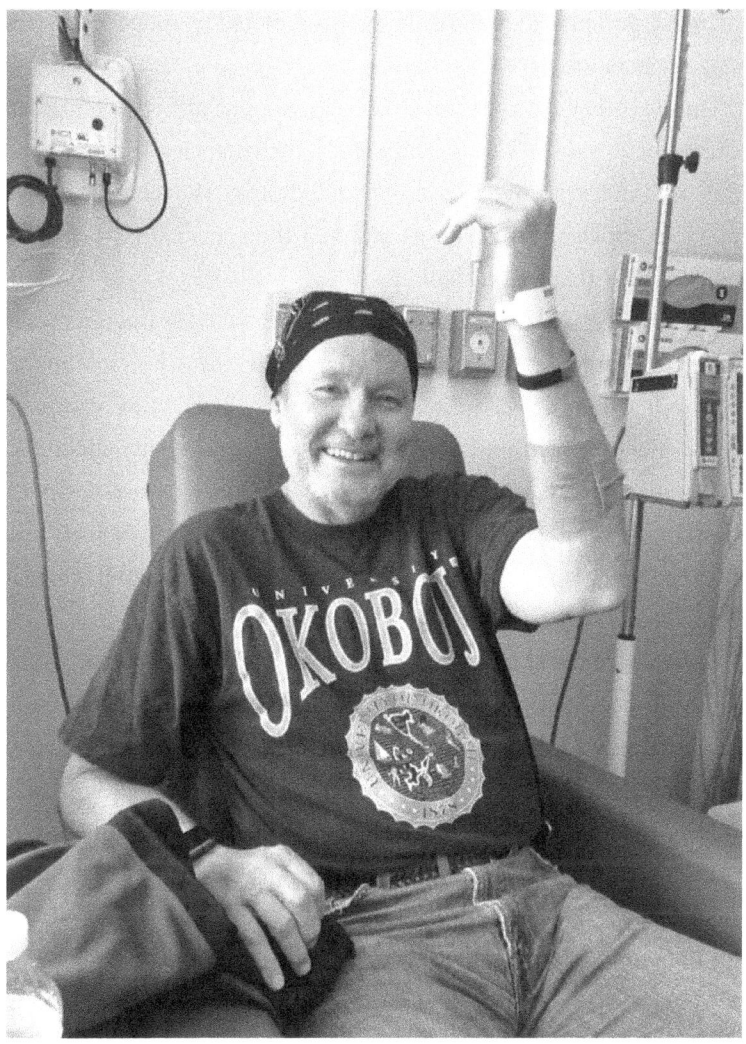

David getting his immunotherapy infusion at Georgetown Lombardi Comprehensive Cancer Center. We'd normally have to sit there for two hours while his treatment took place.

Before 2011, there were no real effective treatments for metastatic melanoma. A small coterie of doctors and researchers had been working unsuccessfully for decades on figuring out how to train the immune system to do its job, that is, to fight the renegade melanoma cells that quickly overtake the body and result in most patients dying within months of being diagnosed with stage 4 melanoma.

Immunotherapy, as it was called, was significantly different than chemotherapy or radiation, which attack malignancies. It empowered the immune system to seek out and destroy cancer cells, while previous cancer-fighting drugs attacked the cancer itself—and too often healthy tissue along with it.

In 2018, Dr. Atkins told us, there were about 1,400 ongoing trials involving immunotherapy and immune therapy combinations to establish which drugs are effective against which types of cancer, and which regimens work best and how to reduce side effects. At the time of this writing, since 2011, the FDA has approved fourteen immunotherapy drugs to treat melanoma in various stages, and doctors were only then starting to build meaningful patient databases.

After decades of trying to learn why the immune system wasn't killing cancer cells as it does bacteria and infections, researchers made a groundbreaking discovery. Cancer cells give off certain signal proteins that deter the immune system from fighting back. Immunotherapy drugs, known as *checkpoint inhibitors*, unleash the full fury of the T cells to annihilate "foreign" cancer cells. A hitch with this theory is that cancer forms from our own tissues, and T cells are hunting for foreign invaders.

Some cancers, including melanoma, have a unique way of throwing up "impenetrable barbed wire" that prevents the immune system, or T cells, from doing its job attacking foreign invaders. Immunotherapy drugs are often able to get the immune system to bust through the barrier and successfully annihilate cancer tumors.

A wonderful irony is that in the worst cancers—melanoma or smoking-caused lung cancer—there are more mutations, making it easier for the immune system to find and attack cancer cells. Side effects are usually minimal, especially compared to the more toxic chemotherapy.

In the Checkmate study David was in, the two drugs (Yervoy and Opdivo) were a unique combination of checkpoint inhibitors that create a potentially synergistic mechanism to help destroy tumor cells. Opdivo helps existing T cells discover the tumor, and Yervoy stimulates T cells to become memory T cells, which can allow for a longer immune response.

Another hitch is that even when these drugs work on a specific cancer, they don't work on *every* patient with the disease. Doctors haven't yet figured out why immunotherapy does not work on all advanced melanoma patients. Those with serious stage 3 (spread to lymph nodes) or 4 (spread to organs) melanoma are put in three buckets: never responders, responders who relapse, and extraordinary responders.

"A lot of research now is how do we decide which category the patient will fall into," said Dr. Marlana Orloff, a medical oncologist in Philadelphia.

Which bucket would my David fall into? We were about to find out.

At first, David's reaction to the treatment was just diarrhea, which was manageable, but once again, my impressive worrying kicked in. I didn't want to call Georgetown about the diarrhea, though they'd instructed us to contact them if there were side effects. I feared David would be kicked out of the trial. Cutter knew I was wrong and reached out to Billy. They let Georgetown know, and we learned diarrhea was a common side effect that's only serious if it went on for days. The diarrhea didn't last, but my flawed judgment indicates how anxious I was. I'm not proud of my behavior as I write this, but fortunately I was surrounded by family with level heads.

However, as time went on, his symptoms got worse.

David is sleeping all the time and generally feels lousy, I wrote in my diary, four days after his first infusion. *He's sick and requires a nursemaid. He cannot take care of himself. I'm having a feel-sorry-for-myself day since this is at minimum a three-month stint. Wah wah. But I love him so much and would be miserable without him. So there's that.*

Trying for balance. Doctors really don't prepare you for the side effects of immunotherapy, other than to list them rapid-fire while you nod. Oh fatigue, check. Well, the guy has been sleeping in twelve-hour shifts, gets up for a few hours, and back down. Hopefully that's because his immune system is in overdrive.

It's so up and down and so eerily familiar to my mother's nine-month battle with smoker's lung cancer, I wrote a few days later. *She was even treated at Georgetown. Initially, she tried chemotherapy and radiation, but the drugs in 1999 weren't what they are today. Nothing worked. The march to her grave was slow and painful, both physically and emotionally. I don't feel built for this a second time around.*

After a few days on our own, Laurence returned to us from San Francisco, as she had a work project nearby. She offered to take David to his first checkup so I could squeeze in time for my writing project.

As she got David out the door and into the car, I was struck again by how amazing she was. She and Billy were newly in love when David was diagnosed with cancer, and she didn't really know any of his family. Yet faced with this crisis, she had quickly become a critical part of the team—calm and empathetic with us, and, I later learned, the shoulder Billy cried on when he was falling apart.

As it got later in the day, though, and they hadn't returned, I began to feel anxious. This time, I was right to worry.

At 6:00 p.m., Laurence phoned me from the hospital. David could barely walk up a flight of stairs without being easily winded. Of the ten items on the list David brought with him of things to discuss with Dr. Atkins, this was the one that got the doctor's attention. Also, his oxygen levels were low. Dr. Atkins thought he might have pneumonia. It turned out that he actually had a virus. When I visited him that night, I had to don a gown, mask, and gloves to enter his room.

On the way home, Laurence asked me again what I was doing to get support. I had no response.

Lying on the bed later that night, though, I thought, *I can't do this anymore on my own.*

Two days later, David came home. That night, I attended my first melanoma support group alone, a group started by Wayne Connors and his wife in Alexandria, Virginia, in 2016.

Wayne was the blogger I'd written to for help when David got diagnosed. He had responded so quickly and positively that it felt like a safe place. I reached out to see if I could come by myself, and he enthusiastically encouraged me to attend.

When I got there, I poured out our story and then started firing questions: "Will he survive? What else should I research? Who should I talk to? Where else should we go?" I was clearly all over the map and in a heightened state of anxiety.

After I finished talking, there was a pause.

"You're such a newbie to this," consoled one member.

"Breathe," said another. "It's a marathon, not a sprint."

They gave me the names of places to get good information, those to avoid ("Dr. Google" being the No. 1 worst), and helped me organize questions for the next visit with Dr. Atkins.

Gradually, as I listened to others' experiences over the course of the evening, it became clear to me that melanoma is a fierce opponent and it would be with us the rest of our lives. By the time I got home,

I knew I'd found a tribe of folks who understood what I was going through.

For the first time in weeks, I felt relaxed going to bed.

A few days later, David was sleeping 24/7, getting up only to pick at food. Laurence had gone back to Philadelphia for work before heading home, and I was by myself again. I went into a second bedroom to have a good cry, lying face down on the bed. Suddenly, I felt a body next to me. It was David. We lay there, his arms around me.

He sleepily said, "I'm in love with you."

He was there, but he was not. *Please come home,* I kept repeating to myself. *I miss you so much.*

By Sunday—Easter—David was as confused as he had been after brain surgery. I knew something was seriously wrong when I found him at 8:00 a.m. washing his hands under the faucet. But the water was off. A friend and I took him to Georgetown's emergency department to get a brain CT scan.

The ER doctor asked David who I was.

"The best," he replied, which brought tears.

He was unable, though, to understand what the doctor meant when he asked David to move up toward the pillow. He didn't know the president's name. Instead of Ted and Billy, he said his sons were Tad and Bully.

The ER doctor said the CT scan showed the brain tumors had grown. I called Billy in San Francisco to tell him the bad news. For the second time in a week, David was hospitalized. The doctor on duty said David was "extraordinarily fragile," and tried to comfort me by telling me about his mother's cancer and how if the immunotherapy didn't work, Georgetown would make sure David was comfortable for his remaining days.

I could barely breathe.

That night, afraid to be alone at our apartment, I called around until I found a friend willing to come over at 9:30 p.m. Billy jumped on the first plane he could, and he and Laurence, who was still nearby in Philadelphia, arrived around 1:00 a.m.

Two days later, David was home again. He had improved, though no one knew exactly why he'd become so confused. Dr. Atkins believed the immunotherapy was working. As the immune system attacks cancer cells, the T cells can inflame the brain, causing it to swell. It's something doctors refer to as "pseudo-progression," meaning the tumors get swollen before they start to shrink.

Over the next week, I watched David like a hawk. One day he'd feel good and I'd be hopeful. The next, he'd say he didn't feel well and my stomach would go into a knot. Was this a bad sign? Was the virus coming back? Was his brain swelling again? He'd been coughing some and spitting up phlegm. I'd listen. I'd count. I'd worry. He'd say he felt like he had a fever and would hunt for a thermometer. I'd offer to rush out and get one. His temperature was 97.6. We'd watch a stupid Adam Sandler movie and he'd doze, later taking a long nap. I'd wonder if this was ever going to end, and how?

That Sunday, I wrote (and then David edited) a blog post for CaringBridge, updating everyone on David's progress. It was, from my point of view, an honest piece of writing. I sent it to Billy for approval. He rewrote it. For the first time, I saw the consultant at work. Rather than an honest, emotional portrayal of what we were experiencing, Billy wrote his assessment—what felt to me like an overly upbeat report. I sent it out as he wrote it.

The next evening, I got an email from Billy.

Lisa, it began. *I know you are doing the best you can. We all are.*

I could feel the "but... " coming.

It did.

Billy was worried about me. More than that, he was worried that my fear was having a detrimental effect on his father.

You and he seem to reflect each other's moods, he wrote. *When you're worried, he's worried. When you're negative, he's negative....To me, the blog that you wrote was an overly negative portrayal of the last two weeks.... It concerns me that this is the view that you shared with him, and it concerns me even more that he agreed with you. I believe his attitude has taken a turn for the worse. This keeps me up at night.... We have all read and heard from doctors and cancer survivors about the importance of a positive attitude, the connection between mind and body. My dad is losing that.*

He went on to tell me to get therapy, lean on support groups, and that I needed to be positive and calm in the face of worsening symptoms.

I felt as if I'd been slapped. His words stung. I was hurt. I got mad at Billy. What was I supposed to do when I did feel negative? Eat it and pretend? This was a tough situation, and my feelings weren't always rosy and upbeat. If he thought I was doing such a lousy job, maybe he could come take care of his dad.

Of course, I couldn't say any of this to David, who was sitting next to me watching TV.

I decided not to respond right away. Instead, I called my friend Terry, a hospice social worker.

She said that was baloney (my word, not hers).

"You get to feel whatever you feel, Lisa," she said, adding that the problem with the belief that people have control over the disease with their attitude was that if the disease progressed, it made people feel responsible, like they didn't try hard enough.

Authenticity and sharing the truth, she went on, were just as important for mental and physical health as a positive attitude.

"This is about you and David talking to each other with respect," she said.

The more I thought about it, the more I talked with friends, my defensive posture receded. Billy was three thousand miles away in San Francisco and scared. I read his email again, and this time other sentences stuck out to me.

I hope you know how thankful I am my dad has someone who loves him as much as you do, who is as loyal to him as you are. No one in their right mind could ask for more than that.... Go to therapy and cry it out (I do it every week).... I would love nothing more than to help search for the best therapists and support groups in your area... Or to arrange for your friends or Dad's family to come down and give you time for yourself... You deserve this.... I don't know exactly what to do....

He was afraid—as was I and all of us who loved David were—that his father might die. He wanted everything and everyone to be okay, and he wanted to help.

And he was right. I needed more support. I needed to share my anxieties with friends or a therapist, not dump them on David. I started going to support groups more regularly. I also went to a doctor to get antidepressants, and that made a world of difference.

7

Reclaiming Our Lives

After his second infusion, David was feeling better. He got dressed and went into his office for four hours—barely two months after surgery. Big milestone. He was still going to speech and occupational therapy to combat the aphasia, but life seemed to be calming down. The drugs caused rashes on different parts of his body, some minor, some not. He was still coughing but not nearly as much, and we were able to do a few four-mile hikes along the Potomac River.

Since David was part of the CheckMate 204 trial to see if his immunotherapy drugs work on brain metastases, he had to have a chest scan and a brain MRI every six weeks. In the middle of May, we took him in for the first set since he'd been home. Dr. Atkins warned us there was likely to be little change. Normally, he would wait longer, but these tests are a CheckMate 204 requirement. They cost us nothing, and the way we saw it, the more information the better.

Yet hours before we were due to meet Dr. Atkins to discuss the results, despite the antidepressants, my hands were shaking. I wrote in my diary:

Trying to remind myself that no news is good news. It means the cancer hasn't grown. And we have had some good news on the lung tumors from the chest X-ray. But really this trial is about whether it works on the brain. Trying to stay optimistic. Naturally, because I'm me, I wonder why they didn't call us to tell us IF it were good news. Seems kind of cruel. I consider it good news that David will get the third infusion this afternoon if the labs look good. I want to get further into this treatment and have more infusions behind us before I can relax.

The news was great. The tumors were smaller. The cutting-edge immunotherapy drugs that doctors—such as our Dr. Atkins had staked their careers on—were working! A different study than the one David was in that would come out in June also had very promising results for us, as David was what doctors call "treatment naive," meaning he had had no previous attempts to get rid of the melanoma.

"Nivolumab (Opdivo) combined with ipilimumab (Yervoy) has high activity in melanoma brain metastases and may be considered for upfront therapy for such patients," said Georgina Long, a clinical researcher from Melanoma Institute Australia, adding that response was highest when given before other treatment. Her study evaluated the antitumor activity and safety of Opdivo/Yervoy in sixty-six patients with melanoma active brain metastases.

A few days after his third infusion, a new rash extended down his back, chest, shoulders, and waist. It itched so much he couldn't sleep, so just after midnight we called the Georgetown oncology hotline for advice. David was put on a six-day regimen of steroids, despite his reluctance since steroids cause him to eat more and sleep less. But he took them, and the rash gradually went away. We wanted to believe this was a sign the immunotherapy was beefing up his immune system, but it could also be that he had an allergy to the treatment. Something else to worry about if it came back.

Still, life was beginning to resume a semi-normal rhythm. David was back at work for a few hours a day, and by his fourth infusion at the end of May, he went for the infusion alone for the first time, and then again alone for No. 5 in mid-June. Dr. Atkins laughed, seeing that David had been allowed to come sans entourage! Usually, I was there at least, and Billy was calling in from San Francisco.

"Clearly the lack of participation in our meetings us one of the prices of our success," David told the doctor.

The June 23 scan showed a near complete decrease in his tumors. And he was back at work full-time. He was doing so well. It made my heart sing.

That same month, before the June 2017 meeting of the American Society of Clinical Oncology (ASCO), a news service that covers the pharmaceutical and biotech industries reported that there were 765 combination drug studies involving immunotherapy drugs in trials on the federal database, ClinicalTrials.gov—triple the number eighteen months previously. The ASCO conference had other good news, particularly this headline in *Science Daily* on June 5, 2017, about the CheckMate 204 trial that David and Dr. Atkins were part of.

"Two combination therapies shrink melanoma brain metastases in more than half of patients." (David was thrilled to learn "his results" were part of the ASCO presentation.)

A few days later, David attended his first melanoma support group. David told his story. He outlined his attitude, how he liked games, and explained his theory of the cancer being terrorists hiding out in his body. It was war he was fighting with diet and drugs, and one he seemed confident he could win. Others in the group listened intently and asked questions about scan results, side effects, and the trial overall. He handled them like a champ. I sat there mesmerized as he talked and wished I had an ounce of his calm positivity. That night, he wowed me.

Maybe Billy was right that I was a bad influence on him.

I knew it was deeper than that, though. Later, when we got home, I was thinking about what cancer was showing us about each other. David and I were built differently and came from different backgrounds. David's father was an alcoholic, and as the oldest kid, he had taken on the role at an early age of holding things together, often with humor and by always having a plan.

I will never know exactly how my father's sudden death from a heart attack when I was eleven affected my psyche, but I do know that there has been a part of me since then that is always waiting for the other shoe to fall. My coping mechanism has been hypervigilance, always looking for the worst outcome—if I can spot it, maybe I can keep it from happening.

Both of these mechanisms had made us who we were. And now, I wondered, were they going to keep us together or force us apart?

David would continue to have side effects from the drugs, but none that put him back in the hospital. It turned out he was allergic to the contrast dye that's injected for CT scans, which caused unbearable itching. This was easily remedied by taking steroids prior to every scan. He also sometimes had canker sores in his mouth that made it difficult to eat anything with spices or even at a warm temperature. He learned to love smoothies. Later, David remarked to Dr. Atkins that canker sores were not mentioned in the long list of side effects of Opdivo.

"It probably will be now," Dr. Atkins responded.

He also sent David to a nose, throat, and ear doctor who prescribed a medicine, tacrolimus, that David could mix with sterile water and swish in his mouth, which took care of that problem. (Turns out tacrolimus was also used by some kidney transplant recipients to minimize immune reactions. Now we wanted his immune system to be strong to fight the cancer, just not in his mouth, where it was apparently overreacting.)

At the beginning of July, we sent out this post on CaringBridge:

July 1, Great news from most recent scans. Last week, Commander Dave was up at 5:30 a.m. to get yet another MRI and full-body scan. We've lost track of how many MRIs the guy has had. No biggie to him. He sleeps in the MRI machine! If anyone has had an MRI, you know that's crazy. The knocking noise is deafening.

I'm burying the lead. "No clear evidence that cancer exists anywhere at this point," Dr. Atkins said this week. Brain tumors have largely disappeared (though the cavities are still there and may be there forever), lung spots remain but unclear if they are cancer. Atkins thinks it is likely scarring at this point given the effectiveness in the brain. Gallbladder is a small fraction of where it started.

The Commander will stay on OPDIVO for at least six more doses and two more scans—another twelve weeks. Then we'll reevaluate. The trial calls for twenty-four months. But this is all so new, often it's game-time decisions.

Commander Dave is thrilled and in charge of kicking cancer's ass...

We were over the moon. We had won, at least for now.

In reading the detailed diary I kept, I'm struck by how quickly, relatively, the news went from annus horribilis to ecstatic in five months. It felt much longer because of the intensity of each decision, each test, each setback, each treatment, each doctor's visit. Such a relatively quick resolution doesn't happen often with cancer, nor even that quickly with others battling melanoma with immunotherapy drugs. We watched another member of our support group, who was treated at Georgetown, go the same route as David, but after two years he died. If we've learned anything, it's that cancer is a particularly individualistic disease and no two cases are quite the same.

With cancer or any serious medical setback, one longs to return to normal or even boring. By fall, we were there. Working. Exercising. Biking. Traveling. David had planned to keep working until he was seventy, but pesky cancer has a way of forcing you to take stock of your life. What did we want to do with our remaining years? David decided he had been handed a second chance, and at the end of November, he officially retired.

That Christmas, we celebrated together with our three sons and their girlfriends and David's ex-wife at Lake Tahoe. It was lost on none of us how grateful we were to have David there, alive and thriving, and wearing his silly Christmas vest.

Good fortune, we would learn, comes in small doses.

8

The Seizure That Ended the Sailing Trip

"I need to talk to you," David said after we got home from a five-hour drive. It was March 1, 2018. The minute he started talking, my heart began pounding, and my ears were ringing. Are there ever scarier words than, "We need to talk"? He quickly reassured me we were fine. It was his health.

"Today, when I was driving back from New York City, I felt a wave of dizziness or mild vertigo that was strong enough I knew I should pull over and let you drive, which I did when it didn't go away in a few minutes," he said.

He'd been feeling dizzy off and on for the last six weeks and experiencing an unfamiliar tightness in his head.

That night, in a restaurant with a friend, I could see David's eyes get watery and feel him slipping away. The dizziness, he said, was happening as I watched. Right away I pushed my quinoa salad aside. He was clearly scared. Once again, I was back to the caretaker role. Trying to be calm on the outside but freaking out inside. When we got home, David and I crafted an email of his symptoms and sent them to Dr. Atkins. Then he went into our bedroom to lie down.

I sat in the other room, looking at the email. *Today is not the first time it's happened during the last six weeks since my last MRI on January 23,* David had written. *In fact, it has happened about five or six times. It started on February 12 when I was driving in California on the highway. It ended very quickly, and I felt it might be something associated with dehydration.*

It's happened five or six times before? I thought. This was the first time I'd heard of this. *And in the last week, it's every day?*

In fact, it happened when I was talking to you and your wife at the Melanoma Research Foundation gala, continued David in his email. *If I am standing when it hits, I need to move my feet around to make sure I am stable, as I feel I might fall over. It seems to be lasting longer, hence my email to you. I should also note that I've recently had a slight headache. Nothing so bad that I've needed to take anything. It's more like a tightness or swelling around my skull.*

I tried to put the pieces together. How had I not known? The month before, we dressed in our best finery and attended the DC Wings of Hope for the Melanoma Research Foundation gala where Dr. Atkins was being honored. Dr. Atkins gave a brief speech about the near-miraculous results of the CheckMate 204 study, singling out David as one of his success stories.

"In oncology, we were taught there was a blood-brain barrier that stops our treatments from working in the brain," Atkins told a packed ballroom. "With these new immune therapies, that barrier didn't exist. One of my patients, who was one of the pioneers who was on that protocol, David Marsden, is sitting over there." There was a loud burst of applause. All eyes turned toward us. "He has just celebrated a year since his horrifying diagnosis of melanoma and is telling me he never felt better in his life." The room erupted in thunderous cheers. David stood up, pumping his fist in the air, Rocky Balboa style, as my eyes filled with tears.

And now I realized that David hadn't been honest. It seemed he was doing what many patients with cancer do when a frightening symptom appears: They wish or explain it away. It was hunger. It was dehydration. He was tired. But now, David, who is not a worrier (that's my job), was genuinely concerned, perhaps even scared.

Dr. Atkins wasted no time emailing back. He suspected that it was the anti-seizure medicine, Keppra, that David had been taking since his brain surgery nearly a year ago. It might be time to start tapering off the Keppra, wrote Dr. Atkins. And with those words, David's whole body relaxed.

But it wasn't the Keppra.

David had an MRI scheduled on March 6. Dr. Atkins was in Paris, so we met with a different doctor. The MRI showed nothing of concern, and it was decided that David would begin weaning off Keppra. Since we were scheduled to leave for a sailing trip in the Virgin Islands the next day, the doctor thought it was better to wait to make any drug changes until after our ten-day trip.

While I'd had more than my share of sailing, David hadn't. He was really looking forward to this trip with our good friends Cathy and Paul and another couple. Paul would be the skipper of a forty-foot catamaran, and we had already put in an order for the charter company to stock it with foods. David spent a small fortune on SPF sun-protective clothing, including a full bodysuit he intended to swim in, to shield him from the intense tropical sun. We both splurged on masks for snorkeling.

The last few days had been frantic. On Sunday, we attended an all-day training to learn how to lobby Congress for more money for melanoma research. Monday, we trooped all over Capitol Hill telling our story to legislative assistants. We got home late that night and began writing the emails we were told to fire off as a follow-up. David stayed up late trying to finish them and clear his plate. He got up in time to be at Georgetown by 7:00 a.m. for his MRI, and I met him at lunchtime for the doctor's appointment.

By now I had taken to downing a Xanax before getting MRI results. David always assumed the results would be good. He was right again. That afternoon, he was cleared for his twenty-fifth immunotherapy infusion!

I sent this text from the doctor's office to friends and family: *MRI results all good* 🐇. *#relieved. Hurrah. Off to Tortola. Can't wait for sailing.* 😊

At 10:30 that night, David was still writing emails to senators. He hadn't even started packing. Nor had he yet taken his evening dose of Keppra. Our flight left at 8:00 the next morning. But he said he could do it all. He'd sleep on the plane.

I was on my laptop on our couch when David got up suddenly from the dining room table. He didn't say a thing, but his arms started contracting like he was a monster trying to scare me. One side of his face contorted. I thought he was trying to make me laugh. He wasn't. He was having a grand mal seizure. I ran to him as his convulsing body fell uncontrollably to the floor, aiming for the thick Afghan carpet.

Foolishly, I put my hand in his mouth so he wouldn't swallow his tongue. (That is no longer the protocol. Instead, you're meant to get the patient on the floor, give them room, put them on their left side. No need to worry about biting the tongue.) He bit so hard on my two fingers that I had bite marks where he pierced the skin. It was a chaotic and frightening few minutes as I pried open his mouth to free my fingers and hit 9-1-1, and then ran next door to enlist a neighbor who helped me get David on his side while the 911 operator calmly talked to me until an emergency medical team arrived. Another neighbor, whom we didn't know, waited in the lobby for the EMTs because we lived in a locked eleven-story building. David stopped convulsing after a few minutes. But it took thirty minutes for him to slowly come out of his trance. It was as though I hit the control-alt-delete button, and he was resetting. To quote Led Zeppelin, he was dazed and confused.

I rode up front with the ambulance driver while David was in the rear on a stretcher. I called a good friend, Chip, who was there at the hospital minutes after we arrived. Cutter talked to me on my cell as we raced through the streets, siren blaring.

At the hospital, they ran tests. But since we'd gotten an MRI that day, I knew the seizure wasn't caused by enlarging tumors. Fortunately, Georgetown had emailed the MRI results that evening, and I could share them with the doctors at our local hospital. The ER doctor told us it was not uncommon for a seizure after brain surgery and, especially, with melanoma meds in the brain.

I canceled our plane reservations and texted Cathy and Paul that we wouldn't be joining them on the 8:00 a.m. flight. David was released at about 5:00 a.m., and we fell into bed surrounded by snorkels, bathing suits, and SPF clothing spread out on the floor ready to be packed.

It was exactly one year to the day that a Hopkins surgeon fished three grape-size tumors out of David's brain.

The next day, after sleeping until after noon, we began scheduling doctors' appointments to figure out why this happened. Even though he was in Paris, Dr. Atkins moved quickly, setting us up with a neurologist who specialized in seizures and brain activity. Two days later, we met with Dr. Tricia Ting, a neurologist who wasn't at all surprised David had had a seizure, even a year after brain surgery. It wasn't the brain meds, she was fairly certain, that caused this; it was more likely a lesion in the left temporal lobe.

"The temporal is a very tricky area," she said. "It tends to make a lot of seizures. Temporal regions are very seizure-genic!" She added, "I don't think it's because the metastases are acting up again and causing swelling and making trouble."

"So calm down!" David said to me.

"I think it's more the aftereffect of surgery," she said. "You have this little nubbin of scar tissue, and under the circumstances—not enough seizure medicine and too much stress—that has built up over time. It just reduced your capacity," explained Dr. Ting.

"What we found in the seizure disorder realm is that taking your time with easing off medicine is warranted," she continued. "People who go two to five years seizure-free do much better than people who go one year seizure-free and whisk the medicine off. We want to keep things quiet. You don't want to start tickling the brain."

Seizures, as she explained it, are an electrical storm. "You have exciting and inhibiting neurons that are kept in balance," she said. "With a seizure, the exciting neurons are stronger than the inhibiting."

The Keppra at 500 mg was used to support the inhibiting neurons to keep the exciting neurons in check. It was possible David *could* have another seizure, so Dr. Ting upped the dose to 750 mg until insurance approved our changing to a newer drug: Briviact.

Her words were a wake-up call. We'd been doing way too much, cramming life into a shoebox as though we were going to run out of time. In the last six months, we'd gone to Arkansas (where I was teaching), the Dominican Republic for a wedding, Lake Tahoe for Christmas, Peru, Los Angeles, and New York City. Sleep had been a low priority. We were guilty of what my ex-husband used to accuse me of: cramming fifteen pounds of @#!% into a five-pound bag.

Time to slow down.

We were forced to abandon biking and switched to hiking on trails outside of Washington, DC. Walking on firm ground felt safer to

David than balancing on a bike, even though he'd been riding one for sixty years. We explored the many trails in northern Virginia, along with River. It helped him feel more normal to be exercising again.

The next issue was an unexpected one, at least for me: David, he of constant good cheer, got depressed.

The seizure represented another front on his war on cancer. He was worried about having another one. He noticed every ping in his head. He was afraid to work out on the treadmill alone, so we agreed that I would go to the gym with him. One day while we were walking to the drugstore, he experienced another dizzy episode. (He'd taken to calling them "dizzy wops.")

"I was just walking," he said. "Nothing out of the ordinary, and then the ground started to shift. I needed to sit down, hold something for support, or at least stop and spread my legs for balance."

He didn't like not being able to do what he wanted. He didn't like being watched so closely by me. He didn't want to curtail plans. I didn't blame him. I wouldn't like it, either.

We headed home and then debated whether to go to Baltimore for a long-planned dinner. I didn't want to go. He didn't want to cancel again. He was pretty down, realizing something was going on with his brain and no one really knew exactly what. And what scared him most was that suddenly nothing was safe.

We went to the dinner in Baltimore and had a good time, but I noticed he was somewhat distracted all evening.

As the weeks went on, he continued to have unexplained dizzy spells. Was it the medication? Or was there something else going on in his brain? We didn't know. No one had definitive answers.

In fact, the dizziness was consuming our lives. David talked about the dizziness all the time, gauging it, measuring it, comparing it to the day before. We were caught in a loop of despair. If I knew the dizziness was related to the medication, I could have relaxed. But because he talked about it nonstop, I worried about it nonstop.

One night, I was sitting in our dining room, and he was standing in the kitchen making tea—a kitchen counter separated us. I looked up to ask him something and he was gone. I screamed his name, ran around the counter where he was lying on the floor. I lunged toward him thinking he was having another grand mal seizure.

"Got it!" David said, calmly getting up.

He'd dropped an almond that had rolled under the stove, and he was trying to retrieve it. It took about ten minutes for my heart to stop pounding.

Me, I'm incredibly anxious, I wrote in my diary that week. *I'm so anxious I can hardly eat. I imagine the worst all the time. I come home, heart beating faster as I open the door and call out David's name and breathe a sigh of relief when he answers. If he's in the bathroom for a while, I call in, "You okay?" I go to the gym with him and stretch to be there to watch him in case he has a seizure. I can't live like this. I can't really focus. It's hard for me to imagine having a real job. Mostly I need David. I need him to be happy, healthy, and in my bed, entwined, every night.*

Two days later:

This morning David wanted to make love. But I was terrified to do it. I was afraid he would have a seizure or a stroke. I am a mess.

Meanwhile David was obsessed with finding out why he had a seizure and worrying about another one. He talked to anyone close to him who would listen, laying out symptoms, concerns, questions. He saw his brain surgeon and asked for a referral to another neurologist (who found nothing), he got our old team (Billy, Laurence, and Rebecca who worked at Johns Hopkins and originally helped us see Dr. Sharfman) together for a call several Sundays in a row to discuss ideas. Finally, Billy rather firmly told him that he had to stop.

"Dad," he said, "you need to come to terms with the fact you are more worried than the doctors are."

In hindsight, it makes sense that after going through all that trauma, the worry would surface at some point.

Finally, we turned to a nonprofit cancer support organization, Life with Cancer. It was a real gift. They offered support groups, exercise, dietary advice, and most importantly, free therapy. Yes, free! I got David to see a therapist to talk about his fears.

This was an expansive time for us.

David slowly learned and then revealed to me that he was most comfortable when he had confidence that he or someone he trusted understood what was going on. Then they could develop a plan. Now there was no plan. He was afraid to commit to doing things we loved doing, such as our trip down the Grand Canyon. After all, if you couldn't count on keeping your balance walking to the store, how could you hike out of the Grand Canyon?

I saw a therapist, too, a woman who encouraged me to get a PTSD appointment. *Post-traumatic stress disorder?* I thought. *Really?* I never thought of that in regard to myself. Then I remembered that when we were in Peru earlier that year on a spiritual trip, the woman leading the group had asked me what I wanted to work on. I said I didn't know; I was feeling pretty good.

And she said, "Really, Lisa? You have been through a tremendous trauma."

Oh yeah, I thought. *I have.*

I'd been so focused on David that I had never thought about my own trauma. After all, he got the life-threatening diagnosis!

But what a life-threatening illness teaches you is that everyone in your immediate orbit is sucked in and suffers and worries along with you.

I brought up David's seizure and his fear in our original melanoma support group, where we went for meaningful help from our "elders," those who were ahead of us in this insidious journey. Missy, the co-leader, reminded me of the need to "adjust your feet, again, to another new normal (the seizure). You can do it," she said. "You did it before, but my experience is that you have to walk through readjusting again and facing grief again."

She was right. I had hoped the worst was behind us, but this was a new chapter in our melanoma journey. It was a reminder that this is not a straight path, which I found particularly jarring since until now, the path had been one of consistent improvement. But that was not the reality with our determined foe.

Once again, as we had when we first started seeing each other, David and I held hands and talked. Who *was* David without his confidence? Who was I without my worry? Both of those things had been coping mechanisms for years, but now they were getting stretched to their limit.

David suggested we get counseling together. He felt we were arguing too much, and it didn't end in laughter as much as it used to. I said no, thinking, *More support? Is that really necessary?*

But David insisted. He'd done couples counseling before and knew it could help. And if there was ever a couple that needed some support, he argued, wouldn't it be two people who were dealing with cancer, caretaking, and managing life after brain surgery?

I still wasn't convinced but finally agreed, in part just to shut him up.

We found a therapist who was a great guide in helping us better understand how the other worked. We began to uncover who we were when we dropped the roles of "the worrier" and "the confidence man."

Of course, being me, I was still skeptical. On many of the trips to the therapist's office, I would be in the car saying, "Do we really need to do this?"

Each time, David would say, "How do you feel after the session?"

I had to admit that I almost always felt better—listened to and understood—and we both got better at listening to each other.

So, we kept going.

9

The New New Normal

Late in April 2018, David went in for a PET scan, a much more expensive, involved test where they inject you with radioactive glucose (called a *tracer*).

Since melanoma, like many cancers, uses glucose to support its rapid growth, it can be identified by the tracers that show up as bright spots on the scan.

Dr. Atkins was on time for our 1:30 p.m. appointment, which was a surprise. Usually, a fellow came in and asked a slew of questions and then would brief Atkins, who would come in later with his nurse, Bridget, for a check. This time, Dr. Atkins walked right in. We quickly got Billy on the phone, and Dr. Atkins asked Bridget to give David the PET scan report and have him read it out loud.

The gist: There were no tumors of any kind to absorb the glucose they'd injected. There was NO EVIDENCE of DISEASE—or, in cancer parlance, NED. As in, David was now NED. Dr. Atkins stopped the immunotherapy treatment. David would come back in thirty days for a "safety" check and then move to a ninety-day appointment cycle where they'd do blood work, MRI and CT scans, and a physical. I cried and hugged Dr. Atkins and Bridget.

David seemed befuddled. He didn't quite know how to react, even though we'd been warned we might talk about stopping the treatment. He wanted to be as excited as everyone else, but stopping treatment was unnerving. It meant we were out on our own. His body was going to have to continue fighting without any help. He relaxed a bit when he realized that he would continue to have quarterly scans and could call Dr. Atkins anytime with questions. But this trial, which called for two years of treatment followed by three years of monitoring was suddenly changing to one year of treatment. He needed time to adjust to this "good" news.

It took me until about 9:00 p.m., when I got home from a work event at the National Press Club, for all of it to sink in.

I walked into the house, took off my coat, and stood in the hallway. *We'd done it,* I thought. *The cancer is gone.*

I went into the living room where David was watching TV. I told him to stand up. Then I hugged him so hard, he could barely breathe.

"Commander David, you won," I said. "Tomorrow night, we are going to celebrate."

For the next six months, nothing happened! At least nothing life threatening. We moved back into my old house, which had been rented, and renovated the bathrooms. David's sons visited for their annual boys' weekend, and I went to the beach with friends. I visited my son and niece Lydia in LA. We made plans for future trips, including trying another sailing trip. We had lunches with friends, went on bike rides, walked River, had dinner together, and watched the news. We argued, consulted, and snuggled together. It was our life together without cancer. And we appreciated it much more than we had before cancer came along.

One night we were in the kitchen having one of our favorite fights—one that took on different forms but whose root was, "Who is right?"

The phone rang. It was Eric, from our support group.

His wife, Joyce, was in hospice.

My heart sank. Joyce? She was so young! Not much older than our kids. It was unbelievable and unfair. Her calm and thoughtful role in our group was a reward for attending.

Eric asked if we would come see her at the hospital. I said yes, of course, and hung up the phone.

"Joyce has gone into hospice, and it doesn't look good," I said to David.

Our argument was over. Being right didn't mean shit when death was this close.

The next day we went to the hospital. Joyce looked like a cadaver, hooked up to an IV and unable to talk much because she had thrush and her throat hurt. Eric was running on autopilot, seemingly in control, not freaking out, and doing what he had to do to take care of the person he loved most. I knew the drill. The breakdown would come later, when he was alone, at the kitchen sink, in the shower, or wherever else it would hit.

I told stories to fill the silence, wishing I... we... were all somewhere else. None of us—not Joyce, not Eric, not her sister, not her brother, not David—wanted to be there. None of us wanted to be in the support group that brought us together. And yet we were, and we clung to each other.

Only thirty-four years old, Joyce would die just three days later. It was a reminder that the beast can always return, and over the next few years, we would see that in action too often. Barbara Lipska, one of Dr. Atkins's star patients who we'd met at a reading from her book, *The Neuroscientist Who Lost Her Mind*, was also having a rough time. At the end of her reading, David had asked a question and thanked her for helping save his life. When David was hospitalized last year with brain swelling from the immunotherapy, Dr. Atkins reassured us that he'd seen this happen with patients (he would never have specified who, but we knew Barbara was one), who had then recovered. Now she was sick again. Later, to our great sorrow, we'd find out that Wayne's melanoma had returned. He'd been on the immunotherapy drug Yervoy, too, but after the third infusion, colitis, a common side effect, was so bad he had to stop and was put on steroids to tame the inflammation.

Why immunotherapy works for some and not others is still not known. Nor is it known why it comes back. But when you're in a support group, you become connected to each other's treatment and survival. Everyone is rooting for everyone else. Everyone wants everyone to win. And then some people lose, and it's a punch to the gut that knocks you down for days.

I was haunted by seeing Joyce lying in her hospital bed, so close to the end of her life. I thought about living in Afghanistan and how death was around me all the time then, too. Not as close and not in the same way, but there all the same. I thought of how despite living with the constant fear of attacks, somehow—amazingly—Afghans remained optimistic about the future. I remembered reading a poll around that time by the Asia Foundation of 9,271 Afghan citizens from all 34 provinces: 79 percent said they were somewhat or very happy. Another 54.7 percent believed the country was moving in the right direction.

I was and still am in awe of their resilience. How did they do it? How do you stay hopeful and find happiness when people you know and love are dying? How do any of us keep living, knowing that other people are suffering at any given moment, all over the world, and half the time we are powerless to help them? Or if we do have power, we're not sure how to use it?

I remembered that back in April 2017, my good friend Kelly Degnan was visiting from Italy. David had just gotten home from a hospital stay, and I was bemoaning the caretaker role. I shared the now-ironic story of how he and I met online and how I had insisted I wouldn't date anyone more than two years older because I didn't want to be a nurse, but there I was, ministering to his every need.

Kelly wisely stopped me and said, "You know, Lisa, the situation could just as well have been reversed with you sick and you would be grateful to have David caring for you."

I thought of how David was always saying he knew he couldn't fix the forest, so he focused on the trees. Maybe that was the most we could do, I thought now… take care of the people in front of us and love them as much as we could. The other thing that occurred to me was that yes, good fortune might come in small doses. Which was even more reason to savor it, celebrate it, and share it as much as we could whenever it decided to grace us with its presence.

10

My Turn

After David was cleared of melanoma in 2017, we wrote a joyous Thanksgiving note to friends and family. The tone was victorious, but the coda contained a caution.

Enjoy the holidays! In fact, enjoy every day. You never know.

Little more than a year later, it was my turn to know.

During the final days of 2018, I was plagued by unexplained anxiety. I had talked about it during our last couples therapy visit. Why was I feeling this now? There had certainly been times in the last few years when David was going through his cancer nightmare when anxiety was called for. But right now, there was nothing I was worried about.

And yet, my stomach was in a knot. By Christmas Eve, the anxiety was so intense I couldn't concentrate or work. I called my internist, Dr. Susan Holland, from a parking lot. She had an opening, and I dashed over. I had seen her three weeks earlier. A nagging cough I couldn't shake sometimes left me feeling like I was running out of air when I was talking. It didn't concern me, though. It was David who'd insisted I have it checked. Dr. Holland had assumed it was an allergy and loaded me up with an antihistamine and an inhaler. It seemed to have gotten better.

Now, after writing me a prescription for Xanax, Dr. Holland said, as I was walking out of her office, "By the way, how's that cough?"

I said that it was still there, but it did not bother me as much.

"Hmm," she said. "Why don't you go downstairs and get a chest X-ray? Let's make sure it's nothing."

I walked down two flights and got in right away for the X-ray. As I was dressing, the technician asked if I was having any pain in my left lung.

"I was last week but not really now," I said.

He asked who my doctor was. "You need to go back upstairs and see her today," he said.

"Is something wrong?" I asked. "You're scaring me."

"I didn't say it was STAT," he said. STAT was the medical lingo for emergency. "Just go see her."

I walked up the two flights, filled with trepidation, and was ushered into a room where I waited alone, fear overtaking me. David didn't even know I was at the doctor's office. I'd expected it to be routine, otherwise I'd have asked him to come with me.

Dr. Holland came in and sat down. "There's a spot on your lung," she said. "We need to do a CT scan." She read the alarm on my face and tried—unconvincingly, I thought—to reduce my panic. "It could be pneumonia or tuberculosis. Or, yes, it could be cancer. We just don't know yet."

I pushed down the panic long enough to book a CT scan appointment for the day after Christmas. Numb and in disbelief, I called David, and we met at a nearby coffee shop. I was experiencing an out-of-body feeling. *This isn't happening*, I thought. *How could a quick doctor visit to get some Xanax turn into a life-threatening disease?* David was, as ever, rational and supportive.

"We will figure this out together," he said. "We'll first get the information. We don't know anything yet for sure."

Maybe my unrelenting anxiety had saved me. I now believe that the mysterious anxiety that had been torturing me was my body or mind signaling that something was wrong, that I needed to see a doctor.

And I was lucky that my internist, Dr. Holland, had insisted on that X-ray. Before being diagnosed, far too many patients with lung cancer go through months of tests and useless remedies (physical therapy, inhalers, allergy medication) for a malingering cough or unexplained back pain before they're finally offered a chest X-ray or CT scan—especially if they're younger or nonsmokers—with the result that lifesaving treatment was sometimes delayed by months. (Note to readers: If a cough doesn't go away after a month, demand a chest X-ray, regardless of whether you ever smoked.)

And I was lucky that I only had to walk down a flight of stairs that day to get the X-ray. If I'd had to schedule it at an outpatient clinic, I likely would have put it off until after the holidays. Then again, Christmas might have been more joyful. Ignorance can be bliss.

On Christmas Day, after opening presents, David, Cutter, and I went to visit our close friends, Cina and Chip, for a family-style Christmas. Cutter and I have spent countless holidays and summer vacations with them in the Outer Banks. They're so comfortable and familiar to me that it was easy to go through the motions. I was somehow able to distract myself from the looming fear—and unspoken certainty—that I had lung cancer. At some point, though, I pulled Cina aside to share my news. *Way to ruin her Christmas*, I thought. But I was scared, and I wanted my friends to worry with me.

The next day, David, Cutter, and I drove to a local hospital for a CT scan. The news was very bad. There was a 4.5-centimeter mass, the size of my thumb, in my left lung. A biopsy was needed, but my internist told us that rarely is anything that size benign. She tried to tamp down my panic.

"We don't know what it is," she kept repeating. But we knew. We knew it was cancer. None of us would say it out loud.

When I asked the doctor if the biopsy would give us the stage, she answered by saying, "Staging depends on whether it is only in your lungs."

She also ordered an MRI. Since the summer, I'd periodically been having bolt-like flashes in my left eye four or five times a month. Dr. Holland didn't think I had brain tumors (if I did, the flashes wouldn't be intermittent), but she wanted a detailed picture of my brain.

I entered a zone of dissociation from what was happening. My whole body was buzzing with fear. I could put one foot in front of the other, I could follow directions, but I couldn't really absorb things or speak coherently.

The plan for that week, before our lives were upended, had been for Cutter, David, and me to drive to Asheville, North Carolina, to be with David's sons and his brother's family for the days between Christmas and New Year's. Should we have the biopsy, or should we go to Asheville? The biopsy can wait, my internist said. Being with family would be a good distraction. I wanted Cutter to spend more time with David's boys. We left for Asheville that day.

For most of my life, when something bad happens, it overtakes me. It's all I can think about.

When my marriage ended, my stomach was in a constant knot, and I could eat nothing but milkshakes. I couldn't sleep without drugs. I wear my feelings like a loud shirt for everyone to see. Rarely have I been able to compartmentalize.

But miraculously I did that week in Asheville. No one said anything to me about the cancer scare or asked questions. It helped that there were a lot of people, big fun family dinners, games, hikes, and other diversions. And Cutter fit in like he'd been coming to these gatherings for years, further cementing the bond David and I had long hoped would form among our kids.

But then it was over. As we said goodbye, David's brother Phil hugged me hard. I don't remember exactly what he whispered in my ear, but I know he was wishing for the best outcome. I felt that in his hug. Among David's four siblings, Phil has always been my biggest fan, often telling me how happy I make his brother.

By 7:00 a.m. on December 31, we were back at the local hospital for a brain MRI and a lung biopsy. The biopsy—a radiation oncologist pushing a needle through my back and into my lung for a sample of the tumor—was painless. But afterward, when I was in the recovery room lying on my stomach, I felt sudden sharp pains around my upper chest and below my heart when I turned over. It hurt so much that it made breathing difficult. I yelled for help.

"I think I'm having a heart attack," I panted. An EKG machine was quickly wheeled in. But everything was fine. The doctor said it was most likely just referral pain, a type of pain that is felt somewhere else in your body than where it originated.

Back home, I rested with a heating pad on my chest while David made waffles for dinner. Cutter decided to hang out with us and watch a movie instead of partying with his friends on New Year's Eve.

The next day, I stayed in bed reading Michele Obama's book, *Becoming*. When my niece Lydia called to wish me a Happy New Year, I drew her into my cauldron of fears, telling her I almost certainly had lung cancer. After I hung up, David gently scolded me, saying I was unnecessarily scaring her. But that was him, believing the results could be good, when I knew deep down that I was right. There was a 4.5-centimeter tumor sitting on my left lung near my heart. I had lung cancer.

Cutter, too, gently tried to buoy my spirits, reminding me how lucky I was to have David and my supportive friends. And to live near two of the best comprehensive cancer care centers in the country—Georgetown and Johns Hopkins. Both hospitals were known for their scientific leadership in clinical and laboratory research and for delivering cutting-edge cancer treatments. I marveled at my son's wisdom and calm. Who was this kid? How did he get so wise?

I knew this was scary for Cutter. He was suffering. I knew how much he loved me. I remembered all too clearly when my mom was diagnosed in 1998 with smoker's lung cancer, how terrified I was of losing her. I kept reminding myself, over and over, a lot of progress had been made since she was treated with chemo and radiation. In fact, OPDIVO, the immunotherapy drug that had saved David's life, worked on some lung cancers. I latched onto that.

Later, I would learn that immunotherapy works best on lung cancers caused by smoking. Smoking-related cells are so badly mutated that it makes it easy for the immunotherapy to find them. Somehow that seemed so unfair, but why be surprised?

Everything about having cancer seems unfair.

On January 2, my internist, Dr. Holland, woke me at 8:45 a.m. She wanted to know if I had an oncologist. As certain as I was of a bad result, I thought, *No! Why would I have an oncologist when I didn't have cancer?* As we spoke, I could barely think straight, so I didn't even ask her how bad it was. She had an opening that afternoon. Could I come in?

A few hours later, David, Cutter, and I filed into Dr. Holland's examination room. She told us that the brain MRI showed multiple lesions, but they were microdots and posed no immediate danger of causing my brain to swell. She couldn't say whether they'd been the cause of the sporadic flashes in my left eye. And she didn't yet have the lung biopsy report, so she couldn't make a definitive diagnosis, but she suspected the tumor was cancer, given its size. Surgery for that was now out of the question since the cancer had spread to my brain.

At least I don't have glioblastoma, a deadly brain cancer, I thought, grasping for some kind of relief.

The three of us stayed in her office for a long time after she left. I cried, and David and Cutter held me, promising we'd get through this. Then we gathered ourselves. I took a deep breath. Something lifted in me. My doctor had said that what I probably had was treatable with radiation. She admitted that she knew little about lung cancer but had read of significant recent breakthroughs. I left her office feeling hopeful.

The next day, I drove Cutter to the airport. He was going to a wedding in Costa Rica. He felt guilty leaving, but he'd already put off his departure once. Now I was trying to be upbeat and encourage him to go and have a great time. That was what a mom was supposed to do, right? Not saddle her kids with her problems. This was going to be a marathon, I told him. I'll need you once we have all the information. As we neared the airport, he started sobbing. When we pulled up to the curb at departures, I hugged him tightly. He was scared. I was scared. There was so much we didn't know.

Back home, I sat waiting for Dr. Holland to call with the biopsy results. It felt surreal to be sitting by the phone waiting to find out what, exactly, was trying to kill me. By the time the phone rang, I was shaking. I put the doctor on speaker so David could hear.

The biopsy indicated that I had lung cancer. My fears were confirmed in two terrifying words. What's worse, it was stage 4 metastatic lung cancer because the cancer had spread to my brain, peppering it with tiny microdot tumors. More specifically, it was adenocarcinoma, a form of non-small cell lung cancer.

Getting a diagnosis of cancer is a huge loss, a shift in your way of being in the world, physically and mentally. Your body has betrayed you. Your world as you know it is gone forever. I didn't know this yet, but a cancer diagnosis would mean constantly trying to claw my way back to that precancer self and never really succeeding. I don't think David feels the same way. He approached his cancer as a problem in need of a solution. He was almost excited to have brain surgery, which would've scared the shit out of me.

Billy called me the night I was diagnosed. We cried together. I told him how upset Cutter was, and Billy said he'd reach out to him.

"We're like siblings," he said, "and if anyone knows what he's going through, it's us."

Cutter told me later that he'd heard from Billy, Laurence, and Ted—each one had called him separately, including his cousin Lydia. After a lot of starts and stops, cancer had truly made us a family.

When I told Lydia, she said that we were lucky. Because of what we'd been through with David's cancer, we knew how to do the research, who to call, the right questions to ask. We knew not to cave in to fear or to go with the first treatment recommendation but to get second and even third opinions. We also knew how to seek out doctors who specialized in certain cancers or in cutting-edge therapies and clinical trials. And we knew which cancer centers in the country were the very best.

"After all," Lydia reminded us, "this isn't your first rodeo!"

No, I thought, *unfortunately it was not.*

I congratulated David. "We now have a platinum membership in the cancer club," I said. "We're a cancer power couple." Even swamped by fear, we were able to interact in a way that could make us laugh or at least smile, as we had done so many times before.

I didn't even know nonsmokers could get lung cancer. I have never smoked cigarettes in my life, save for sucking experimentally on a few Tareytons or Kools in high school. But research shows that up to 20 percent of people who develop lung cancer have never smoked.

What's more, the actual incidence of lung cancer in people who have never smoked is increasing. No one is certain why this increase is happening, or how much of it might be because as the number of smokers in the United States declines, the proportion of patients with lung cancer who smoke will also decline.

I'm part of a growing lung-cancer cohort known as never-smoked women. Women are much more likely than men to get lung cancer if they have never smoked—more than twice as likely. The reasons are unclear.

There are different types of lung cancer. I have been diagnosed with non-small cell lung cancer (NSCLC), which is the most common type, accounting for about 85 percent of cases. Small cell lung cancer (SCLC) accounts for about 15 percent of cases. It is a more aggressive, fast-growing cancer that is mainly caused by smoking.

As I reeled from the news of my diagnosis, I dove into the statistics. The five-year survival rate for NSCLC was 25 percent, compared to 7 percent for small cell lung cancer.

I will be the exception, I thought. *I will be in that 25th percentile.* As I read on, however, I learned that for cancer that has metastasized and spread to other parts of the body, as mine had, the five-year survival rate was terrible. Only 7 percent made it that far. I reminded myself that these statistics were already out of date; stats online are always out of date. If a figure of 7 percent was based on the last five years, it didn't account for the most recent developments in cancer treatment.

I tried to employ my mantra, refined during David's cancer: *Ignore the statistics.* And yet they always found a way to burrow in.

How did this happen to me? I thought. I couldn't stop searching for clues. In our bedroom, on top of the heavy mahogany dresser—something I inherited from my mother—was an 8 × 10 black-and-white publicity photo of my mother from her acting days on TV. She looked stunning. I saw it every morning when I woke up. Mostly, it brought me comfort. But now, in the wake of the diagnosis, I was filled with rage. *You did this to me!* I thought. *You caused me to get lung cancer.*

My mother smoked filter-less Chesterfields every day, year after year, for more than sixty years. I can still see her long, regal, black-and-gold cigarette holder. I grew up hating smoking, passionately, something I told her many times. At some point, I even made up a rhyme about it: *My mother smoked everywhere, near and far, and always in the car.*

My mother smoked from the age of nineteen until she was eighty. I can still recall the fetid smell of overflowing ashtrays in my childhood home, which filled me with disgust. I can remember rinsing them out, the putrid odor of water mixing with cigarette ash. I remember riding in our Ford station wagon and my mother throwing her arm across my chest—no such thing as mandated seat belts then—to keep me from sailing into the windshield when she had to stop suddenly. The irony is that our car was always filled with deadly cancerous fumes.

I spent a lot of my childhood trying to bat cigarette smoke out of my face. It caused me to cough and choke. Now I think I should've tried harder to escape it.

My mother had started to smoke back when smoking was common, but as scientific evidence of the dangers of tobacco mounted and smoking became less socially acceptable, my mother's world shifted. She became a pariah. We had some wicked fights when I was in my thirties and forties, when she would visit my home and I'd refuse to let her smoke indoors. One Christmas when I exiled her to the front porch of our friend's house, so angry about her smoking that I didn't care that it was freezing cold, she slipped on the icy steps. We only discovered her accident when she didn't return and we went out to check and found her lying in her mink coat in the snow, dazed but unhurt.

Still, she lived to be eighty-two. She was diagnosed with lung cancer at age eighty-one. I was sixty-five when I was diagnosed, and

I will likely die from it at a much younger age than my mother did. It never seemed fair that she got more years of life than I did, and I had never smoked.

How could you do this to me? I would think, accusingly.

I couldn't say for sure, of course, that she did do this to me. While researchers can connect smoking to squamous cell carcinoma and small cell lung cancer, adenocarcinoma—the type of NSCLC that I have—is linked to multiple potential causes, including genes, indoor and outdoor air pollution (burning wood, coal, kerosene), radon exposure, family history, and other factors.

For thirty years, I have lived in a house built in 1918. Though all types of houses can have levels of radon, a hazardous gas, older homes are thought to be more susceptible. A radon test of our house was inconclusive. For two years, I worked in Kabul, where people commonly burn tires and plastics for heat, and the weather report is sometimes "smoky."

Or *was* my mother to blame? NSCLC has also been linked to secondhand smoke. But I grew up at a time when nearly everyone's parents smoked. If my cancer were solely secondhand smoke, a lot more of my contemporaries would have lung cancer.

When I was diagnosed, I had no bandwidth to be angry at my mother. That would come later. Sometimes my anger flared; other times I was more forgiving. Eventually, I would make my peace with her. My mother didn't know how dangerous secondhand smoke could be; no one did back then. Now, the U.S. Surgeon General estimates that living with a smoker increases a nonsmoker's chances of developing lung cancer by 20 to 30 percent.

"Even brief secondhand smoke exposure can damage cells in ways that set the cancer process in motion," according to the Centers for Disease Control. "As with active smoking, the longer the duration and the higher the level of exposure to secondhand smoke, the greater the risk of developing lung cancer."

I certainly never dreamed that I could get lung cancer from the clouds of smoke enveloping my childhood. As an adult, I'd been healthy, athletic, an exercise fiend. *If I don't smoke like my mother*, I'd thought, *I'll be okay.* But as I came to know, "If you have lungs, you can get cancer."

11

We Can Help You

With one terrible phone call, the roles David and I had been playing had just flipped. Now, as my caretaker, he was typing furiously at his standing desk, preparing questions for my first doctor's appointment. I loved him so much as he jumped right in to help me.

A cancer diagnosis can either strengthen or destroy a romantic relationship.

The challenges we were facing would test our relationship in ways we couldn't foresee. But we would do this cancer together, just as we had the first one.

My first consultation with an oncologist was a bad fit from the start. Driving to the doctor's office as a certified patient with cancer, I was virtually catatonic, unsure what to expect, and once again, filled with fear. Fortunately, my neighbor Celeste offered to drive us and employ her medical expertise.

Dr. S. asked me how I was feeling. I responded that I felt great and considered myself a high-energy person always on the go, forever busy, that the cancer hadn't slowed me down. The day before, David and I did a twenty-mile bike ride. She noted that on her pad.

Then began a physical examination, with me on the table, and David and Celeste seated nearby. As the doctor was listening to my lungs, she commented, "You don't strike me as a high-energy person."

I burst into tears. I said I was terrified. That might account for my lethargy. Later, I told a friend about her odd observation, and he replied, "You have to wonder how many bubbly new patients this oncologist meets? Perhaps aberrant mental health in America walks through her door routinely."

I should have walked out then. She possessed the empathy of a rock, though that insults rocks. Yet we let her convince us that, given the microdot tumors in my brain, I should have ten days of full-brain radiation and needed to start right away. She made an appointment with a radiation oncologist in her practice, who we saw the next day.

Given all we had learned about potential long-term damage from David's brush with brain radiation at Hopkins, I wasn't keen on the idea. Yes, we knew radiation was effective, but it could do a number on one's ability to retain information and often does long-term damage to short-term memory. The radiation oncologist said, for example, I might go to the grocery store for five items and forget two. Never mind that I would lose my long, blond, thick hair, which my hairdresser has always marveled over.

"The hair gods were very good to you," she liked to say.

Since none of us has control over their hair—you get what you're born with—I took it as a compliment. Later, I'd lose my hair anyway as the cancer progressed.

As we'd done with every doctor's visit, we recorded the appointment and shared it with our in-house medical team. Billy and Laurence listened to the audio with Dr. S. They were not impressed. They noticed I was impassive in the meeting and only stepped up at the end when Dr. S. suggested full-brain radiation and I strongly voiced my concerns. Later, David met with our full in-house medical team. Before those who weren't there had a chance to criticize, David told them, "We didn't handle that well. We let Lisa take the lead and she wasn't prepared to ask the questions we need to ask. Next time will be different."

The second doctor I consulted was Dr. Stephen Liu, the director of thoracic oncology at Georgetown's Lombardi Comprehensive Cancer Center. David emailed Dr. Atkins the minute my internist telephoned with the diagnosis. Eight minutes later, Atkins responded with an appointment with Dr. Liu.

David and Celeste went with me to the appointment at Georgetown, the same place my mother had been treated unsuccessfully for smoker's lung cancer in 1998. I popped a Xanax to calm my nerves.

When Dr. Liu walked into the cramped examination room, he ignored my companions, took my hands, looked directly into my eyes and said, "It's generally my practice to be very upfront about things. I want to make sure you understand that we can't cure you, but we can help you. There's going to be a good treatment for you."

I hardly needed to hear more—I was going to live! It was true there was no cure for stage 4 lung cancer. But clinical trials in the last five years had led to more treatment breakthroughs with lung cancer than in the previous twenty years and, in some cases, could turn lung cancer into a chronic disease. In the past, so few survived stage 4 lung cancer that it was only recently that survivor groups had formed to advocate for more money for research and how to thrive with cancer.

I chose Dr. Liu as my primary oncologist. It was an easy decision.

In the following days and weeks, I amassed more knowledge than I ever wanted about my kind of lung cancer. I did a deep dive into lung cancer research (surprise!), taking webinars, listening to podcasts, scouring the web and periodicals for studies and articles on the topic. My first shock was learning the data about how many people get lung cancer without ever smoking and how many of those are women.

In fact, lung cancer diagnoses overall have risen a startling 87 percent among women over the past forty years while dropping 35 percent among men over the same period, according to the American Lung Association.

To me, the increase in women seemed like it must be tied to genetic or hormonal differences, given that's a distinct difference in the sexes. Studies over the past few years suggest that estrogen may promote the growth of lung tumors, which may account for the earlier age of diagnosis in young women.

In 1987, lung cancer surpassed breast cancer to become the leading cause of cancer deaths in women. But there was some good news: People were living longer.

"When I started in this field nearly twenty years ago, people with advanced lung cancer were living six to twelve months after diagnosis. Survival rates today are significantly improved," said one of the doctors I followed, Dr. Alice Shaw, director of thoracic oncology at Massachusetts General Hospital in Boston.

Medical advances in diagnosis, targeted drug treatment, and immunotherapy are changing the field radically, and at a breakneck pace, but I think there should be wider adoption of early screening. Even though lung cancer in nonsmokers is known as the "silent killer" because it presents few symptoms until it has progressed to stage 4, only smokers or ex-smokers are advised (and covered by insurance) to get screening chest X-rays for early detection. If you can get regular routine mammograms and pap smears, why not routine chest X-rays or CT scans?

In the months to come, as I adjusted to my new reality, David schooled me on the ins and outs of scheduling MRI and CT appointments at Georgetown, who to call, what paperwork was needed, and so on. It was like he was my older brother, and I was starting high school.

"Don't leave your books in your locker. You won't have enough time between classes to get them."

When I told him this, we burst out laughing. We were in this mess together... again. Sometimes I'd catch him looking at me the way I used to look at him when he was in the throes of his disease. Checking, all the time.

Was he okay? Was he eating enough? Had he taken his meds? Did his eyes look funny?

Now he was watching me.

Just as they had for David, our actual families stepped up, surrounding me with love and support, listening to the recordings David and I made of our meetings with my doctors, discussing my options. We recorded the meetings because I needed to listen to them later at home when my heart wasn't racing and I could concentrate.

I felt so blessed, so *not* alone in my ordeal, surrounded by love and people who wanted me to beat this. I remember being struck by a comment one time during David's treatment when several of us crowded into a Georgetown examination room. A nurse remarked how lucky David was to have such a supportive family. I thought that odd. Doesn't every patient come in with family?

"No," she said, "no, definitely not. You are unusual."

All awkwardness between David's boys and me was long gone by then. When I emailed Billy from the waiting room one day, neither of us thought twice about saying how much we loved each other.

Me: I could not love you more, Billy. Thank you for listening to the tape so quickly. As you could tell in Dr. Liu's manner and voice, he's a gem. No question where I'd go. Georgetown in a heartbeat.

Billy: Dr. Liu is a gem. But you know who's the real gem? You!! Lots of love. We're going to figure this out!

12

The EGFR Jackpot

If I had been diagnosed with stage 4 metastatic lung cancer a few years earlier, I would have automatically undergone the standard treatment of chemotherapy or full-brain radiation. Lung cancer was regarded as a single disease, and chemo was usually the one-size-fits-all treatment. The side effects were brutal, and the prospects for survival were measured in months, not years.

Instead, Dr. Liu ordered two types of biopsies—one that took a bite of my tumor, which would be sent to the Mayo Clinic for detailed genetic testing, and another that involved a vial of blood. The blood would be scrutinized for bits of DNA the cancer cells had shed into my bloodstream. The blood test could detect alterations in a panel of fifty-five genes linked to multiple cancers, without the need for a biopsy. It would determine whether I was eligible for a targeted cancer pill that I would take once a day.

According to Anne Chiang, MD, PhD, a Yale Medicine thoracic medical oncologist—another doctor I came across while doing my research—treatment was getting more specialized.

"We used to think all lung cancers were the same, but now we understand that there are different kinds. The good news is that the types of lung cancer that nonsmokers tend to get are usually driven by a molecular change or mutation that can be detected in the tumor, and there are drugs and therapeutics available for them."

If there were certain mutations, or biomarkers, found in my tissue or blood, my cancer could be treated with a pill. *A pill!* No chemo. No radiation. No hair loss. No nausea. Just swallowing one pill a day. Cutter and I would marvel about this, laughing a little nervously: Shouldn't there be an IV drip involved? Would I be getting off too easily?

Biomarker testing has revolutionized cancer treatments. After the Human Genome Project was completed in 2003, it gave researchers the DNA reference blueprint, identifying many actionable genomic alterations, meaning there is a pill to take depending on the mutation.

Since NSCLC is a genetically diverse disease, biomarker testing provides valuable information for a lung cancer diagnosis. Lung cancer biomarkers, also known as *tumor markers*, are biological molecules in people with lung cancer. They can tell how aggressive a cancer is, what kind of treatment will be most effective, and whether an individual is responding to the current treatment protocol. This kind of testing can come from blood or a biopsy or both. Depending on the results, it might mean no chemo, which I dreaded.

"Biomarker testing is so important in lung cancer today," Dr. David Carbone of the James Comprehensive Cancer Center at The Ohio State University told me. "A patient who would otherwise get toxic chemotherapy and have an expected survival of less than a year instead lets your doctor select an oral, nontoxic therapy with medium survival measured in years."

There are different names for this testing, but the most advanced type of sequencing technologies is called next-generation sequencing (NGS), "which can test for hundreds or thousands of genes in a single test," said Carbone.

Unfortunately, not all oncologists run this special blood test when a patient is first diagnosed. Too many doctors go straight to prescribing chemo, especially when patients are often treated by a general oncologist in a community hospital setting.

Less than half of patients with lung cancer are given a comprehensive biomarker test, according to my doctor and other research. As a result, a large percentage of patients are not given the opportunity for a targeted therapy. Why is unclear. In one 2021 study, those patients with lung cancer who got biomarker testing also had medical insurance coverage, access to the tests, and were treated at elite clinics.

If you receive a lung cancer diagnosis, the very first thing you should do is make sure your doctors have ordered comprehensive biomarker testing done on your lung cancer tumor.

Like ovarian cancer and some other cancers, NSCLC is usually discovered at a late stage. More than 80 percent of lung cancer diagnoses are stage 4, as mine was, so it's important, in my opinion, to go to a National Cancer Institute—Designated Comprehensive Cancer Center or other academic institution—to be genetically tested and seen. There are only seventy-one Comprehensive Care Centers in the United States, located in thirty-six states. Fortunately, I lived near Georgetown University's Lombardi Comprehensive Cancer Center.

As of 2021, there were fourteen biomarkers identified for potential targeted therapy lung cancer treatments, according to the Lung Cancer Foundation of America.

But not all of them can be treated with a pill. Currently, there are nine mutations with FDA-approved targeted therapies for lung cancer. Mutations where targeted therapies exist are much more likely to occur in patients who never smoked. That is what is meant by "targeted therapy" or "precision medicine." The treatment is tailored to my specific type of lung cancer.

Each type of targeted therapy works a little bit differently, but all interfere with the ability of the cancer cell to grow, divide, repair, and/or communicate with other cells. Targeted drugs can also limit damage to healthy cells. (Chemotherapy can be effective, but it can't distinguish between healthy cells and damaged cancerous cells.)

Precision medicine is based on the premise that each of us is biologically unique, and we therefore need bespoke drugs to battle our cancers. Matching the right treatment to the right patient has dramatically improved outcomes, with more patients with stage 4 lung cancer living longer with a cancer that used to kill them within a year of diagnosis.

At the time of my diagnosis, the odds of someone having one of the commonly known biomarkers were 15 percent, but it was even higher for a female never-smoker. Dr. Liu said there was likely a 60 to 75 percent chance—or even higher—of my having a treatable mutation. He suspected I had the epidermal growth factor receptor (EGFR) mutation, which was the most common mutation that is targetable. About 10 to 15 percent of those diagnosed with NSCLC have the EGFR mutation.

"Nobody wants to have lung cancer," said Dr. Natasha Leighl, of Princess Margaret Hospital in Toronto. "But the truth is, that if you're going to have lung cancer, EGFR lung cancer patients have the most hope. It means that people with EGFR-positive lung cancer have a real chance to have targeted therapies, to avoid chemotherapy, and to live longer, and to live better lives."

I wanted to have EGFR. As a fifteen-year-old, I wrote to my mother that *I never wanted to be ordinary.* I still have the yellow handwritten four-page letter that only an idealistic teenager could write. My mother kept it and passed it on when she was dying. When I wrote it, I was away babysitting for the summer. I was full of ambition and told her I had only two goals: to be strong and to be intelligent. *I want to learn, to travel, to comprehend life, to know more about religion, its history,* I penned in print. *God is created out of man's fears. I need God to help me and so I pray, but why can't I pray to Zeus or the door?*

Now I tossed all that grandiosity aside. I wanted desperately to be conventional, average, to have the most common mutation. If I did have it, the pill used to treat me wouldn't cure the cancer, but it would likely shrink the tumors and cut the signal that was instructing my cancer to grow, like a breaker switch cuts the electricity. The pills would also work on the microdots of cancer in my brain. Just days before, another oncologist had recommended ten days of radiation without even waiting to find out if I had any mutations.

Reminder to readers: Always get a second, even third, opinion.

Three days after my appointment with Dr. Liu, he emailed me to see if we had heard any news about the tissue biopsy sent to the Mayo Clinic. He reached out several times to Mayo and checked on my blood work.

Research has shown that a caring, empathetic doctor can make a difference in health outcomes. These caring gestures won my heart.

A week or so after the tests, I was coming home on the Metro subway from a conference in DC when David called me. Dr Liu had given him the good news. I had the EGFR mutation! I'd hit the jackpot, if a terminal disease could have a jackpot. Patients with EGFR-positive lung cancer may have the most hope of survival. I wanted to shout *Hurray!* on the crowded subway, to share my terrific news with the other riders. Instead, I breathed a sigh of relief.

Doctors have known about the EGFR mutation since 2004, when investigators at Dana-Farber Cancer Institute in Boston discovered that a subset of lung cancers showed mutations in the EGFR gene, a finding that helped catalyze the field of precision medicine for patients with lung cancer. EGFR is a protein that lives on normal cells. When this protein is turned on, it signals this cell to grow and multiply. A mutation (or change) in a gene can create an abnormal protein on the cell and that leads to the abnormal protein telling the cancer, "Grow. Grow. Grow."

Paul Kalanithi, the neurosurgeon and author of, *When Breath Becomes Air*, had EGFR lung cancer. He died in 2015 at age thirty-seven.

Four months later, AstraZeneca's drug Iressa was approved as a first-line treatment for metastatic NSCLC with the EGFR mutation. Another EGFR-targeting drug, Tarceva, had been around for more than a decade by then, but the science had only recently progressed to allow doctors to identify which patients would benefit from it.

I would take Tagrisso, a third-generation drug that attacks the EGFR mutation, which had been approved by the FDA less than a year before my 2019 diagnosis. It worked better than previous generations of EGFR drugs. (I didn't have the right biomarker for immunotherapy, so chemo and radiation were backup options.)

Tagrisso had been particularly effective in advancing "progression-free survival," meaning it stabilizes and slows the growth and spread of the cancer. It had a downside, but it wasn't the side effects, such as sudden diarrhea or rashes, which I considered minor though inconvenient. It was that no one could predict how long Tagrisso would stave off the cancer's growth. Given how different our bodies are, it might work on one person for six months and on another for three years. Still, I felt lucky to have it.

I began taking Tagrisso the following week.

13

Losing Judy

One day when I was about ten years old, I was snooping in my mother's kidney-shaped mahogany desk and found a packet of letters on blue stationery, bound with a rubber band and addressed to Judy Burns. My older sister's name was Judy Shepard. Naturally, this got me curious (a trait that would benefit me greatly later as a journalist), and I read one of the letters. It was signed, "Love, Dad."

When Judy got home, I asked her about her two surnames and found out my mother had been married before. It was a big emotional scene with a lot of tears. Judy hadn't wanted me to know we had different fathers. She was sure that if I did, I wouldn't love her as much. (She was wrong.) And now that I knew, she never wanted me to mention her father again.

My relationship with Judy was complicated. She was thirteen when I was born. When I was a toddler, she took me everywhere—even on dates, I was later told. I was her doll, her toy, and she was my dazzling, drop-dead-gorgeous big sister. I was one of her bridesmaids when she got married at twenty-six, and I was godmother to her first child, Courtney. She was the most generous person you could meet, and she loved me fiercely. But I think something had happened to Judy when she was young, before our mother married my father in 1950, which my parents either didn't know the details of or wouldn't say. Whatever it was seemed to have left a well of insecurity that Judy spent her life trying to fill.

For a time, she lived a great life in San Francisco—big house, expensive cars, country clubs, a ranch in Napa. But in 1987, her second husband was killed in an attack in a bar in Solvang, California. It upended her world, and she never recovered from it. Her husband had left a trust fund for the kids' education and more than $1 million to Judy. She burned through that money, and by the time she was in her sixties, the rest of the family was helping her out. I resented it—I'm realistic and sensible, and I had saved assiduously and planned for my future—but I never stopped sending her money.

But there were two Judys, and the other one was generous and kind. When I shared my cancer diagnosis with her, she told me she would pray every day for me until I got better. I swear she would die for me, if given the chance. When there was a positive development, she texted, *I love you so much. Your good news is my good news.* When I told her how expensive my new drug was going to be, she said that as soon as she'd paid off her bills, she would give me whatever money was left. At the time, she was in the midst of a years-long lawsuit against an ophthalmologist who had left her blind in one eye. The lawsuit was finally scheduled to go to court. Despite endless legal setbacks, she'd persisted, and I told her how much I admired her for that.

Judy herself was very sick at the time of my diagnosis, extremely weak and in horrific pain. She'd become very difficult by then, demanding complete fealty from her family members; anything less was, to her mind, a betrayal or attempt to hurt her feelings. Being around her was like walking on eggshells. And yet she could also be loving. My feelings about her, it's no exaggeration to say, were complicated. I loved her. I felt sorry for her. I wanted to help her, but she made it frustratingly difficult.

On the day I was to begin taking Tagrisso, the phone rang at 9:00 a.m. in my Virginia home. It was Lydia, Judy's daughter, and she was hysterical. She was incoherently blubbering about my sister, Judy. *Judy's dead.* What? I bolted upright out of bed and begged Lydia to slow down and start from the beginning. My heart was racing so fast that it pounded in my ears, making it even more difficult to understand.

Lydia's older sister, Syida, spent the night with Judy, who had recently gotten out of the hospital, though none of us thought she should have left. Judy insisted on being discharged for reasons not worth explaining. She'd been hospitalized with a prolapsed anus, something people don't normally die from. She was feverish and almost delusional when Syida got her to bed. Syida had tried to enlist the support of Lydia and their brothers in getting Judy back to the hospital. But my sister protested vigorously, so the kids agreed to wait and see how she was in the morning.

When Syida went to wake my sister that morning, Judy was cold and stiff. Dead.

Once I got the story out of Lydia through her tears, I hung up, stunned. David had left for a breakfast meeting. What does one do when her sister, who practically raised her, dies unexpectedly and one is three thousand miles away? I sobbed in the shower. I called my brother Jay, followed by a flurry of phone calls with family that offered no greater understanding. Only passing on the shock.

I muddled through the day in a stupor, still wracked with tumors in my lungs that were making it increasingly more difficult to breathe. At this point, I could barely do anything without labored breathing. My back was going in and out of spasms that only got worse after my sister died. I had spent too many days lying on a heating pad, loaded up on pills, to quiet the spasms and dull the pain, afraid to move.

That day, January 29, 2019, should have been a special day. After my ad hoc medical team and I decided on Dr. Liu as my primary doctor, he prescribed Tagrisso, which retails for—are you ready?—$15,785 a month out of pocket. I wrangled with my insurance and paid $2,614 for the co-pay (after that, it would be $980 a month). It's ridiculously expensive, but it would save my life, so it was a bargain. And I could afford it. Later, I learned that the manufacturer, AstraZeneca, has a financial assistance program, for which I was eligible based on my age and retirement income. Later, I got the drug for free.

That night, I took my first dose of Tagrisso, a small, pinkish, oval pill that *should* prevent the cancer from growing or spreading, and works well reducing or eliminating tumors in the brain. Before I swallowed the first pill, I offered a prayer of gratitude out loud to the scientists, researchers, doctors, trial patients, and to AstraZeneca for this chance at extending my life. I said a prayer for all my predecessors with lung cancer who didn't live long enough to benefit from this miraculous drug. I was overwhelmed by the incongruity, the feeling that for me to live, my sister had to die. I know it makes no sense, but it haunts me still.

14

Who Am I with Cancer?

Within five days of starting on Tagrisso, I started feeling miraculously better. I was less winded walking up the thirteen stairs to our bedroom. The cough, which had been getting worse—I sometimes coughed so hard my head ached—was easing. I began to feel like my old self, though my energy was still low, and the painful back and shoulder spasms persisted. My physical therapist said that with all the emotional stress, my autonomic system had sent my body into red alert. A life-threatening diagnosis and my sister's sudden death had overloaded my system. It would get better, she promised, while working my shoulder muscles. And it did, as I gradually accepted my new normal. The absolute worst had happened. My lifelong fear of cancer had become a reality, and I'd lost someone important in my life whom I loved.

A month later, David and I met with Dr. Liu. I told him that if I didn't know my lungs and brain were riddled with tumors trying to kill me, I'd say everything was fine, I was just a little out of shape.

Dr. Liu was confident the Tagrisso was working. He scheduled brain and chest scans to see what was happening. He expected the tumors in my brain to be smaller, maybe even gone. It was still a little too early to see a maximum response, he said, but we could find out if we were on the right track—whether this was the right drug. Meanwhile, David and I had already paid for a seven-day rafting trip through the Grand Canyon in April that involved hiking out seven miles, with an elevation of one mile, to the Canyon Rim. I wondered if I could still do the trip. Dr. Liu not only approved our adventure, but he also encouraged me to do it. Hiking out of the Grand Canyon at age sixty-five with stage 4 lung cancer would turn out to be one of the toughest, most rewarding things I've ever accomplished.

But first, we needed to be sure that the cancer wasn't growing. In mid-March, after scans of my chest and brain, we met with Dr. Liu again.

Tagrisso was the right drug.

Only a small circle of close friends and family knew my secret. Over the weekend, David and I biked twenty miles with neighbors I've known for decades, but I said nary a word.

"Cancer is not something that makes you want to share," said Suleika Jaouad, a young woman with leukemia. "It's something that makes you want to hide."

This is exactly how I felt. I didn't want to share this news at all. It was hard to tell people. Mentally, though, I was struggling with the diagnosis. Shortly after I was diagnosed, I had sent an email to a select group of friends who I called my Fuck Cancer Kitchen Cabinet. I explained what few facts we had, ending with:

What I need you all to do is get down on your knees, send positive thoughts, do a rain dance, scream at the moon, meditate, or perform some special voodoo. I am not telling anyone other than who is in this group. So please do not share this information without my permission. I know. Unlike me. But that's how I feel. Much love, Lisa

When David was diagnosed in 2017, I couldn't keep my mouth shut. I was so distraught that I burdened anyone who would listen.

But me, my cancer, no way I'm telling the world.

Telling someone you have cancer can be difficult, it says on CancerHealth.com. *There will never be a perfect time to share this news, and often, people worry this information will place a burden on those closest to them. These barriers—difficulty, timing, and guilt—may sway people to avoid the topic entirely, and instead try to deal with a cancer diagnosis privately.*

This was very out of character.

I'm one of the most public people I know. I post picture after picture on Facebook, documenting my latest travel adventures with David. I'm a reporter. I thrill to see my name in the newspaper. I love teaching, appearing on TV, speaking in public, writing personal essays. I'm the first up on the dance floor making a fool of myself.

There were a handful of times when my younger self might've stripped off her shirt while dancing. My fifty-year-old self might have done something similar at her birthday party.

David was certain I'd botched my chances of getting a security clearance in 2014 while I was being vetted for a possible government job after I wrote an op-ed in *USA Today* critical of US intervention in the Afghan presidential election. (I got the job.) I'm certain I didn't get a security clearance with the ultra-private Aga Khan Foundation because there was too much of me on the internet. If you met me on a plane, I'd likely chat you up until I got the essence of your life story.

But keeping the cancer news to myself was a way for me to hang on to a sense of power as my world was spinning out of control. My body had betrayed me, just as David's had betrayed him. His way of controlling things was to stick religiously to an anticancer diet, cutting out red meat, dairy, sugar, white rice, potatoes, and only drinking Pinot Noir, because it has the most resveratrol, which is said to have anticancer and anti-inflammatory properties. Mine was to control the flow of information.

There were other deeper reasons I safeguarded who I told—some simple, some worth exploring. The first highlights the paradox that comes with a life-threatening diagnosis.

I've witnessed this over and over and can find no way around it. You share devastating news, and the minute the words are out of your mouth, you are bombarded with questions, most of which you have no answers for. They love you. They are scared, too. The news is stunning, shocking, overwhelming. They are in such disbelief that it becomes *your* responsibility to comfort and reassure them. It's an odd but real phenomenon.

I didn't want to tell people because I knew it would upset them and require me to make them feel better! Sometimes it took more psychic energy than I had.

I remember waiting until we were halfway through lunch at a restaurant before I got the nerve to tell one of my favorite people. "I've got some news," I said, spilling out my story. Her fork, heavy with salad, stopped midway to her mouth as though she couldn't fathom eating. I jumped in, words tumbling out, reassuring her, my hand on her arm. "I only have to take a pill. I am going to be okay. I have a great doctor. David is the best. We just biked thirty miles. I am not going to die." I comforted her until I saw the fear in her face relax. And yet she continued to stare at me, dumbfounded—just as I'm certain I would do if a good friend told me what I was telling her.

I surprised another good friend who'd been a lifesaver when we both lived in Afghanistan. We had almost finished our meal where we'd talked about David's cancer, our dog, mutual friends, work, writing… everything but me, my news. Each time I decided to tell someone face-to-face, I found I had to steel my courage, put the best spin on it. When I told Jean, she gasped. I had mentioned I was thinking of writing a book about our cancers.

"If you do, you should title it, *Oh, By the Way, We Have Cancer*," she said. "I can't believe you waited until now to tell me."

The irony is that they should have been comforting me. But this experience was so consistent that I found it easier to say nothing. Upon hearing my news, a survivor-friend of throat cancer texted me wise words I keep close:

Lisa, I just wanted to reach out and let you know I am thinking about you. As one cancer survivor to another, my advice is laugh, cry, throw things, love your family, and if anyone tells you cancer is a gift, tell them to fuck off. Do cancer however you want to do it—privately, publicly, laughing, crying, whatever works for you. There is no right or wrong way to do it. But listen to the Drs. and do what they say. And don't piss off the nurses. They are the ones that do the hard work.

But the other reason for my reticence, which was harder to admit, was that cancer was not how I saw myself. It wasn't supposed to be this way. I had planned to live into my eighties, doing yoga every day. I didn't want to get put in a cancer box, like it was my new ethnicity. I didn't want to be defined by it. I was still the same person; I also happened to have cancer. I didn't want my cancer to be the first thing that comes to mind. If I was struggling up that hill on my bike, huffing and puffing, most people would think it's because I have cancer. With a world that's clueless, if I was panting up a hill on my bike or during a hike, it was because the hill was steep and I'm sixty-five! I didn't want people scrutinizing me for signs of my illness. For now, swallowing a pill with few side effects allowed me to look and be like everyone else, that is, normal.

Maybe it all went back to hating the way people looked at me after my dad died. I clearly remember to this day, when I was a tween, friends saying to me about weekend plans, "What do your parents say?" and quickly correcting themselves. "I mean your mother." I was the only one I knew who didn't have two parents in suburban Montclair, New Jersey. I didn't want their pity. I wanted to be like them and not be defined as "child of a single parent." We weren't like the "normal" families surrounding us, with dads commuting into New York City and moms home to greet us after school. If I were going to stand out, I wanted to do it on my terms—not theirs.

As it may now be clear, I've worked at cultivating a persona of someone strong who can handle whatever comes her way, as someone brave, adventurous, fearlessly independent. It's how I've approached my job as a reporter: fearless. It's how I've approached life. As someone who wasn't going to let cancer keep me down, I wanted to get a text just like what a Fuck Cancer Kitchen Cabinet friend, Cathy Trost, unwittingly sent when I needed it the most:

I was just thinking so strongly about you when your text came through. I don't want to demean what you are going through with platitudes. But I've always felt like you are one of the bravest, toughest people I know. You don't back down. You don't take "no." You are physically strong and fearless. Your courage is fierce. Let's take this Mother/F DOWN.

Cathy's portrayal of me, honestly, was a well-cultivated, decades-old facade. There was some truth to it, but thinking about it as I write this, it was more like a costume I liked to wear in public, a favorite jacket I knew looked great on me. I didn't let many people see me in the moments when I took the jacket off, when the cancer reality would sink and I'd fall down a rabbit hole of fear and anxiety. I was afraid that I'd suffer, that I'd have the same screaming pain my mother had, where only morphine eased her discomfort, though there was never enough. I was, and still am, afraid of dying, of leaving behind all those I love. But I kept those fears to myself.

All of this begged a larger question: If I stopped trying to prove how strong and fearless I was, who would I be? Why couldn't I have cancer and be fearless? Why was I afraid of making myself vulnerable to the world around me? Why did I fear pity? Why didn't I share my fears with my friends and close family? Was I in denial? Likely so.

The only close friend who opened the death door was Tara Brach, a friend from high school who lived nearby. She came over one day, and while holding my hand, said, "You can talk to me about anything. I've thought a lot about death and mortality."

Most of my close friends couldn't bear to think of me dying. Some said it. They only wanted to hear good news, which I would reciprocate if they had a terminal disease. Accepting and delving into death and what it means was hard for me.

What I wasn't doing was allowing myself to be vulnerable, which I can see now hurt not just me. Holding back, not admitting I was scared, was denying the people who loved me the opportunity to step up.

Without vulnerability, there is no human connection, says lecturer and best-selling author Brené Brown, known for her studies on courage, vulnerability, shame, and empathy. She spent years interviewing study subjects who were comfortable with vulnerability. She concluded that people who experienced more joy and love were people who were willing to be vulnerable. Which to me meant doing things like saying I love you first or telling those closest to me I was scared.

Still, I didn't want to share my fears with my son, Cutter, or my niece, Lydia. I knew they loved me very much and depended on me, and my cancer frightened them. I held back, too, from my closest friends, always trying to put the best spin on a recent setback.

Maybe it wasn't fair to them. Maybe holding back was denying them opportunities to be there for me. But I also felt like it was allowing us to skirt the elephant of death that lived in the center of our lives.

Fear of vulnerability, I now realize, is what made me hold back from embracing the early days when I first met David. I feared rejection, heartache, shame, embarrassment. It felt safer to stay on the sidelines, but David didn't give up on me, and for that I'm grateful. With cancer, I'm not worried about losing David or him rejecting me; I'm confident he's my greatest support.

A week after my diagnosis, one of my best friends, Judy Belk, who lives in Los Angeles, came to see me. I brought David along to our dinner because I knew he'd temper my catastrophizing. When Judy got back to LA, she texted:

I know you are getting ready for a battle, so think of me as one of your foot soldiers ready to help you fight in any way I can. Assume you know you have a cute, loving man by your side. It warmed my heart to see how much he loves you in big and small ways. I know you won't take that for granted. I love you.

What I am afraid of is dying, which is where I feel most vulnerable, and alone, and I don't talk about that with Judy Belk or really anybody. When I share my fear with David, he rationally responds that we all are going to die, we just have more information. My closest friends are there, but I can't bring myself to talk about my fear of death. Talking makes it too real. (It was Cutter who said, "You can't feel brave without acknowledging some fear." He still surprises me.)

I expressed a fear to my therapist, Micheline, that I didn't want to burden David and Cutter with caring for me when I got near the end, like I had to do with my mother in 1998. It was painful to watch someone I love slowly die and give up all hope that she would get better. It all took a toll on my marriage and on Cutter, I could see now.

Micheline had a counterpoint. Maybe David and Cutter and anyone else would *want* to take care of me and comfort me.

Yes, I thought later. It had been a gift to take care of my mother, to see her through the nine months to the end of her life, to be there as she took her last breath. Why had I assumed that caring for me would only be a burden for the people closest to me? Later, when I got sicker and had to start taking chemo, friends were begging to come take care of me. But by then, while death was still a taboo subject, asking for help became easier—if only to take the full burden off my wonderful David.

Once, we got into a bind when I had a treatment the same day that David was scheduled for a medical procedure. He needed someone to drive him home. The perfect person was his good friend, Paul Magnusson, who had had the procedure a year before. But then Paul got sick and David had to find someone else. His friend from work, Chris Payne, appeared honored to be asked and happy we thought of him. This was, for me, a new perspective. People wanted to help us. They wanted to cook meals for us, to grocery shop, to run errands.

I knew that I couldn't choose which emotions to feel, numbing those I didn't like and then expecting to feel fully the pleasant ones—like being blown away at people wanting to help us. If I numbed myself to fear, I also numbed myself to joy. I was looking for certainty in an uncertain world.

But there are no guarantees. So I started sharing more of the things I had kept to myself. I told Lydia I knew there were no treatments to save me, that it was now all about just buying more time. I told David to let the people in our neighborhood bike group know why I was not showing up for our weekly rides. And I found the more I let people know what was really happening, the more I was able to feel their love.

They say cancer changes you, and it does. What cancer has unleashed is my daily sense of gratitude and joy in little and big moments. I focus on those, whether it's sitting around a firepit with my son and his girlfriend, Diana, who we both adored, laughing with David over something silly, or hiking along the Potomac with friends. I take none of it for granted. David too. He radically changed his diet; he dedicates himself to exercising and making the most out of every day. He knows if it were not for breakthroughs in immunotherapy, he would not be here.

About two years ago, we bought former ABC weekend anchor Dan Harris's app "10 Percent Happier," a meditation guide that offers fifteen-minute meditations that we do each night together, and I can honestly say it has changed me. I try to be patient anytime I'm on hold for a long time or unable to reach a doctor. No one is being intentionally rude, and even if they are, I figure it has nothing to do with me. In other words, we would later learn, we had begun unintentionally practicing mindfulness. I didn't rush from event to event; instead, I worked at being present as much as I could rather than living in constant fear of a future where I would die. I decided to live. I noticed the trees in the spring as they began to bloom, and how my garden grew daily in the summer, rather than hurrying by, oblivious to the beauty around me. This would become more and more difficult as the cancer progressed and my fears exploded, taking over my daily life.

15

The Grand Canyon

One morning in early March 2019, David asked if I wanted to go to the quarterly melanoma support group through Life with Cancer, a local nonprofit dealing with all cancers and their concomitant issues. I said no. We already attended a different melanoma group that we had joined when he was diagnosed in early 2017. Those are our people. I was not interested in yet another. "Besides, it's Wednesday night," I told him.

David: "What are we doing Wednesday night?"

Me (jokingly): "That's the night of my lung cancer support group. You know, you aren't the only one with cancer, Buddy. I have it, too. And I have my own support group."

We started laughing. I was lying in bed, having just woken up. He'd been up for hours. He jumped on the bed and started tickling me!

I felt lucky to have him but got annoyed—yes!—at his chart on the refrigerator to measure how many cups of water I'd drunk each day. My nutritionist said I needed to drink eight to ten glasses a day. My water bottle counted as two. He wanted to know how I'm doing on protein. I needed eighty grams a day, and that could be tough. I found Siggi's yogurt! One serving has fifteen grams of protein. Two of them are thirty. Booyah! I told him in therapy one week that I wanted to be in charge of my eating and drinking. He was hurt, I sensed.

It was my life on the line. Of course, I'm going to pay close attention to what I eat and follow the nutritionist's suggestions.

During the early months after my 2019 diagnosis, Billy and Cutter were both visiting. One night I came home and the three of them clearly had been talking. They asked me to sit down at the kitchen table. My heart began racing, but it slowed when I realized this was a dairy intervention! My three men—and I silently reminded myself love motivated them—didn't think I should consume any dairy. Billy believed it caused inflammation. Cutter was down on it, too. And David had been off dairy since he began his anticancer diet in 2017. I naturally, not surprisingly, got defensive, arguing that my nutritionist was encouraging me to eat cottage cheese and yogurt and drink milk—not soy or almond.

To defuse things, David played an earlier recording when we met with the nutritionist. Our sons concluded she wasn't a quack, and I agreed to meet with her so we could discuss the dairy conundrum that would go on for the next weeks and become a topic for David and me to discuss with Micheline, our couples therapist, at our next appointment.

When we met the next day with the nutritionist, she was clear that she wanted me to strive for eighty grams of protein—how I got it there was my choice. She explained the research wasn't conclusive that dairy was bad for you. But if they felt strongly, there were ways to get to eighty grams without milk, yogurt, or cheese. I felt somewhat bullied but didn't speak up. I reluctantly agreed to cut out dairy. I did what I too often do. I shut down, not being honest about what I was feeling in order to make them go away. What I should have done was said, "It's clear that you guys love me and want the best for me. But I need to think about this and come to my own conclusion, and I hope whatever I decide, you will support."

This issue came up several times more and earned the appellation of The Great Dairy Intervention. Gradually I came around, giving up cheese, switching to pea milk, and adjusting my diet on my terms. But that was before I lost my appetite and got down to a weight I hadn't seen in decades. Then I ate yogurt, whole milk, and cheese again.

But I had a much bigger challenge looming: our Colorado River rafting trip through the Grand Canyon. Dr. Liu had given me the go-ahead. But was I strong enough? Rafting might be relatively easy, but the trip ended at Phantom Ranch, where we'd leave the rafts and hike out of the Canyon—seven miles up to the rim! I was strong enough to take spin classes and work out with machines to increase my stamina. Cutter was still around to train me, and he had me walking fast, panting up a nearby steep hill.

We arrived in Flagstaff, Arizona, in mid-April, nearly missing our connecting flight due to airline screwups. Had we not made the flight, we would have missed the entire trip. Rafting through the Grand Canyon had been a lifelong dream. Rafting in April on the Colorado River was a trip of a lifetime. It was so quiet, so still, so overwhelming, when mile after mile there was absolutely no sign of civilization. I was humbled that these steep canyon walls were exactly as they were in 1868 when John Wesley Powell rafted down the Colorado. Powell traveled these same waters with hunters, trappers, and fellow Civil War veterans. The canyon was just as it was three years ago, thirty years, three hundred. We were surrounded by red and gold cliffs, moving through aquamarine, heart-attack-cold water. At one point, on a dare, David jumped into the freezing cold water. He could not get back in our raft fast enough!

The trip sailed by, and in my inimitable way, I'd stashed my fears about the upcoming hike deep in my duffel bag. They were real. All the rafting company literature warned this was a difficult hike, not for everybody.

"If you and everyone in your party lives an active lifestyle, vigorously exercises multiple times per week, enjoys a physical challenge, and hikes often, the Bright Angel Trail will be doable for you," warned the rafting company's website. The five-thousand-feet-in-elevation hike might not be for you if you have asthma, a history of heat-related problems, take meds that dehydrate you, have heart disease, vertigo, balance issues, fear of heights, are overweight, smoke, are out of shape, or are old! "Be honest to yourself about your current physical capabilities," it said.

Nothing about lung cancer. I wanted this challenge.

We rose at 5:00 a.m. the morning of the hike. There were six of us, and I knew I would be the slowest. We'd hired mules to ferry our duffel bags to the top. All David and I carried were day packs filled with water, snacks, and peanut butter and jelly sandwiches, the latter of which we ate at Indian Gardens, about halfway up the Bright Angel Trail. We refilled our hydration packs with fresh water at one of the few stops on the trail. A guidebook suggested the hike would take anywhere from six to ten hours. The two twenty-nine-year-olds got out in four hours. I took the longest, clocking in at eight hours. Another couple our age made it in five or six hours.

David easily could have finished it in five hours. He would hike ahead and then wait for me. I plodded along with a guide, Helen Rainey, that our rafting company had sent to accompany us. Her job was to stick with the slowest hiker. Me! Helen knew from the required medical forms that I had lung cancer and could not have been kinder, encouraging me to keep putting one foot in front of the other under the burning noonday sun. The views were breathtaking. But I could barely enjoy them during the steepest last quarter of the trail, where I had to rest every three minutes to catch my breath and get my heart rate to slow. We'd been advised that when you huff and puff, your body doesn't get enough oxygen to function efficiently. If you can talk while you walk, that's the right speed. But there was no way, when it was nearly vertical toward the end, that I could walk and talk. Sweat streamed off me, my shirt soaked and baseball cap rimmed with a salt line. The last portion was brutal, but no way was I giving up.

At the top, Helen snapped a picture of the victorious, exhausted couple, arms around each other, hiking poles defiantly raised. Without stage 4 lung cancer, this would be a feat deserving bragging rights at age sixty-five. The fact that the cancer didn't prevent me from achieving a dream was a gift.

We collected our duffel bags and headed to the Maswick Lodge, where we'd spend two nights at seven thousand feet. I'd been dreaming of cold shower and clean clothes. The only bathing we'd done in the last week were quick dips into the icy Colorado River. I never had the nerve to get my hair wet. It was heaven to wash out the sweat and dust caked into my shoulder-length blond hair.

After a forgettable meal, we slept the sleep of the dead. Until about 5:00 a.m. I woke coughing like I did before I started taking Tagrisso.

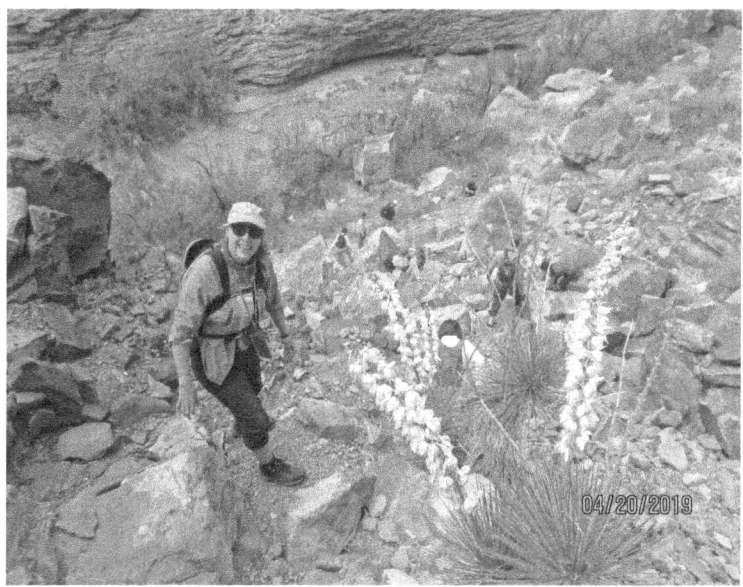

Hiking in the Grand Canyon. Ultimately, we hiked out 9.5 miles with a 4,380-foot climb from the bottom to the rim. I was determined to do it and proudly did.

Was the cancer back? For the next few hours, I could only sleep half-sitting-up between cough bouts. I panicked and emailed Dr. Liu:

For most of today, when I'm vertical I don't cough as much. But I am quickly winded walking up the one flight of stairs to our hotel room. I'm hoping it's the altitude and exhaustion. I really taxed my lungs Wednesday and am concerned by how quickly I get out of breath here. I didn't imagine my lung capacity was so limited. Could I have damaged them on the hike? David, on the other hand, sprung up the trail.

In addition, I get easily cold, chilled, then feel hot, and like I have a head cold with my glands tender. Feel sleepy. Not sure if it's a cold, exhaustion, elevation, or it means the cancer has already outsmarted the Tagrisso. How does one tell the difference between a cold and cough and a cancer-has-returned cough?

Dr. Liu responded in a few hours. It wouldn't be the last time he'd have to talk me down from the ledge. His response was short: *I feel confident you will feel much better when you get down to Phoenix.* And he was right. As we dropped down in elevation driving to visit David's older brother, Carter, in Phoenix, I could feel my lungs opening. I was breathing as easily as I had as we moved swiftly along the Colorado River. The next day, my birthday, I slept all day.

I was victorious. But how long would I be able to take on such feats?

16

Scanziety

David and I got scanned up the wazoo every three months. We'd get snapped in and delivered into big, white, hulking, donut MRI machines whose sound penetrated our chests, abdomens, and brains, searching for traces of cancer, measuring tumors to the millimeter, looking for new growth. The noises for this hour-long procedure would be so loud, a technician would put foam earplugs in my ears to dull the thud, thud clanging.

My doctor told me that he often holds his breath while waiting for a patient's scan to load, hoping to find nothing changed.

David eventually stopped the scans when his doctor declared him in remission on March 9, 2021. Before he left Dr. Atkins' office that day, he asked how he should answer the question, "Do you have cancer?"

"You can say it's in remission." At four years with clean scans, Dr. Atkins said there was no more than a single-digit percent chance of it *returning*.

David and I did cancer differently. Our situations were different. While immunotherapy had melted away David's tumors, with my lung cancer, there would always be something to measure. The best I could hope for was that things remain stable.

For me, it was a matter of not "if" but "when" the cancer would outsmart Tagrisso. And it would. As miraculous as my Tagrisso was, it would stop working. Doctors use the term *progression* (though it sounds like something positive, it's not) for the time when the cancer outsmarts the drugs and starts growing again. At that point, we'd go to Plan B, which would be determined by whatever the latest developments are in lung cancer treatment.

But our temperaments were also very different. David assumed his results would be good. In the interim between scans and results, he slept like a baby and didn't waste time worrying.

I was not built that way. That short window of time—a day or two at most—was treacherous for me. My state of mind, known in the cancer world as "scanziety," was consumed with what-ifs. I looked for signs everywhere. Before each scan, I was certain the results would be bad. I'd come up with little mantras to reassure myself: If I made it through this green light, my results would be good. If I could hold that plank for one minute, there would be no new growth. I thought certain examination rooms were good luck—though I could never remember which ones when I arrived for my scans.

David and I even had opposite ways of enduring the scans. Once, while waiting for an MRI, I opened my eyes and realized that my head was immobilized in a locked cage shaped like what baseball catchers wear. I freaked. It was all I could do not to squeeze the red "panic ball" in my hand. Claustrophobia, I repeatedly told myself, was not an emergency. David, on the other hand, could fall asleep inside the deafening jangling and clanking of an MRI machine. He pretended he was going off in a spaceship traveling deep into outer space.

Once, I tried visualizing during a CT scan. I thought of all the people who loved me and cared about me and wanted me to do well. They floated in my mind, and I could feel their love and warmth. But then I thought, *Wait, the only thing that would bring all these people together would be my funeral.* I tried to laugh it off and focus on all the positive energy.

These days I pop a Xanax thirty minutes before scans. And I *never* open my eyes.

Even now, as I await my results, I tend to spiral, imagining the worst. Is the slight wheezing in my chest a warning sign? Am I coughing more than usual? Is the cancer back? Feeling healthy is no comfort. Cancer is sneaky, as David and I know.

We'd both been largely oblivious to what was growing inside of us, almost up to the day of our diagnoses. I focus more on cancer stories.

Once, I read about an American couple living in New Zealand who had been forced to move back to the States because her drug, Tagrisso, wasn't covered by insurance in New Zealand. She looked like me; she had the same cancer. The couple had sold their home, cars, and boat and left adult children behind. I had expected it to be an insurance story, but the story was about the woman dying—after her last scans had been clear. How could it have happened so quickly? When cancer starts growing again on Tagrisso, it's supposed to grow slowly.

I tended to read and join everything related to my cancer. Some were helpful. Some, like the previous story, were not. But I read one now-forgotten article and managed to save this quote that I read as scan time came near:

It's possible that everything is going to be okay. To me, it holds more options—it might mean I have cancer for the rest of my life, but it's also possible that everything will be okay within that context.

After my diagnosis in 2019, I joined a Facebook group for people with my EGFR mutation. At first I found it helpful, but then it seemed that only the people who were in trouble would post, and I felt myself dragged down with them. For over a year, I'd stayed away from the group, but somehow (thanks, Facebook), sporadic posts from this group started reappearing on my feed. One night while waiting for my own results, I read about a husband who'd held his wife's hand as she took her last breath. As anxious as it made me, I couldn't seem to look away.

When the day of the scan results arrives, I'd go to the waiting room and pace or sit tapping my foot rhythmically like a metronome. When Dr. Liu came in and gave me the all clear, I felt like a prisoner on death row who'd just gotten an eleventh-hour reprieve. I'd take a deep breath, smile broadly. I could go back to my life, leaving my cancer anxiety at the hospital for the next three months. Now, after endless consultations, tests, and doctor's appointments, doing everything possible to fight off the cancer, I'm now in the acceptance phase. From here on in, it will be maintenance. Quarterly scans. And watching and waiting.

The new cancer therapies have given both David and me extra years of life. But for patients like me, these treatments have also created a limbo state of wondering whether my cancer will return before the next advance in treatment arrives. I noted in my diary:

I know I should feel grateful and I am. I'm going to focus on staying healthy both mentally and physically. Struggling a bit now with the mental part. I'm scared.

When I go to a dark place, which I've been doing lately, I think, *I'm lucky if I'm alive in two years.* When I break out of it, I know that if I feel good and can live my life as I was before the diagnosis, it's easy to stash the truth in the closet. Yet every time I meet with Dr. Liu for the results, I wind myself up so tightly and get so tense, I'm like a rubber band stretched to its breaking point.

In September 2019, David and I biked to Georgetown to meet with Dr. Liu. Cutter gave me a pep talk the night before about staying positive going into the examination room. The time before that, I bit off the nurse practitioner's head when she had begun asking me the usual routine questions before Dr. Liu came in.

Nurse Practitioner: "Do you have pain anywhere? Do you have any diarrhea?"

Me: "Yes, I have it right now. But it's because I'm so nervous about the scans."

Nurse Practitioner: "Oh, I'm so sorry. Your scans are good. All clear. I'm sorry I didn't say something sooner."

In this way, I lurched mentally and emotionally from one scan to the next. I no longer shared my anxiety with David because he finds my reaction so foreign.

For most patients with cancer, the longer they go without the cancer recurring, the greater the chances that it won't return. But that's not true for patients with stage 4 lung cancer. It works in reverse. The cancer will return. I know it's crazy, given the reality of the disease, but I try to trick myself into optimism. It wasn't like tiptoeing past a graveyard but more like moving toward it, while believing your luck won't run out, that you'll never actually get there.

I'd read enough to know that trying to suppress fear doesn't work, it only amplifies it. Harvard psychologist Susan David counsels that acceptance of our emotions, including the negative ones, is critical to developing resilience and achieving true happiness, not just the shiny "model patient on a pedestal variety." I knew I needed to dive "deep into the suck," as Dr. David wrote, and face what might happen: I could run out of treatment options, experience the pain my mother did, and die much sooner than I wanted to. I couldn't pretend that I didn't have these feelings, but I could learn to manage them and not let them rule my life. It ain't easy, though.

With practice, I slowly learned that diving deep and identifying the monster lurking in the shadows (e.g., "I am feeling fearful that I will run out of treatment options, experience pain, and die sooner than I would like.") was key. It was scary initially, but facing it led to palpable relief. Much better than tiptoeing around the shadows and settling for a false positivity I couldn't trust, as my friend Terry had told me back when I wrestled with Billy's email on my impact on David.

Once I could name what was hiding in the dark, it was easier to see how much good there was around me, and I could focus on that and live a life filled with gratitude.

I'm still not sure what to do with my fears when they are peaking. I'm sure that I won't be around next year, or maybe the year after that. I have a terminal disease. There is no cure. Someday I will run out of options.

When Billy and his wife, Laurence (they married in 2019), confided they were pregnant in 2021, they asked me what I wanted their son, Finn, to call me. I said I had some time to think about it and would get back to them. In my head, I was thinking, *It doesn't matter. I won't be around by the time their son starts talking.* I hoped I was wrong.

17

C797S and the CyberKnife

In spring 2020, David and I were living in San Luis Obispo, California. I had a three-month gig as a visiting journalism professor at Cal Poly, and we were exploring the area, equidistant from our kids in San Francisco and Los Angeles, as a potential retirement spot.

We were there when COVID-19 hit. Three weeks before we were scheduled to drive home, California went into strict lockdown. Overnight, San Luis Obispo, a thriving college town, turned into a ghost town. But as the death toll began to climb, we decided it was safer to stay there than drive back across the country, not knowing what we'd find or where it was safe to overnight.

Every day, we hiked or biked for miles. It was awesome to hike up the rolling hills and dunes, to see and hear the ocean. One day we hiked up Valencia Peak into the fog and as we came down, the Sun emerged, illuminating the fields of wildflowers. Another day we biked twenty miles to Pismo Beach. It was hard for me as an extrovert to isolate during the lockdown, but I was grateful to be living in a place where I could lose myself in the beauty of the outdoors. If you had to be stuck somewhere during COVID, this was pretty good. I never wanted to leave.

Then in May, I began experiencing pain in my right leg, which got steadily worse. I could only sleep on my left side. I was sure it was exercise-induced. I worked virtually with my physical therapist and then saw a chiropractor. But the pain was becoming excruciating. I never thought to connect it to cancer because I'd had my routine chest CT and MRIs in mid-May and had been given another three-month reprieve. What I didn't know was that the CT scanned only my lungs. A tumor would have shown up if the CT scan went down to the bottom of my spine. I'd wondered if the pain was related to the hip implants I'd had in 2012 and 2013. Whatever it was, I was in can't-sit-still, moaning pain.

By June, I was emailing my oncologist in DC, Dr. Liu, begging for medication to thwart the pain. But Dr. Liu's medical license prevented him from prescribing most narcotics in another state, so the best he could offer was Tylenol with codeine.

I desperately tried to get an appointment with my orthopedist in Palo Alto, who years ago replaced both my hips. We traveled to Palo Alto for X-rays, but they showed nothing wrong with the implants. The doctor ordered a full-body bone scan and an MRI of my spine. And he gave me a prescription for oxycodone. Bless him.

As I sat at the Palo Alto Medical Clinic a week later waiting for the results of the scans, I wasn't worried. I figured I'd be told a herniated disc was the cause of the pain running down my right leg, which by now was under control with oxycodone. Given that we were in a pandemic, hospitals and medical offices are not allowing family members to accompany patients to appointments. David, my rock, couldn't come with me. We did have a plan. He'd drop me off and then drive to our friend Megan's house. I would call him when the doctor came in, so David could participate and record the visit.

As it turned out, I should have been worried. My doctor wanted an X-ray, so I left my phone in the examination room and went off with a nurse, leaving David hanging on the line. My doctor came in, saw the phone, and asked David to come back to the clinic. He would waive the COVID rules. That's when I knew I was in trouble. David sped back over to meet me.

"There's a tumor pushing on your L3 vertebrae that is pinching the sciatic nerve and causing pain," the doctor said. "I'm going to get in touch with your oncologist and see what he wants to do. I'm so sorry. I know this isn't the news you wanted."

There was also a small tumor on my left shoulder, a spot on the middle of my left arm, and a spot on my skull. I was stunned. While David asked the doctor questions, I cried.

Within an hour, Dr. Liu called from DC. By then, David and I were sitting by the pool at our friends' Megan and Peter's house in Palo Alto. Dr. Liu explained that the cancer had figured out how to grow outside the EGFR pathway by "opening a back door," another way of saying the cancer had become resistant to the drug.

"So, the way we manage this is by trying to figure out which back door they've opened and see if there's a way we can close that door. Now, this is obviously a lot earlier than we had wanted. But we're prepared for that, okay?"

I'd been on Tagrisso since January 2019. We knew this would happen eventually—Tagrisso is effective, on average, for nineteen months before patients develop resistance—but it had happened a lot earlier than we'd hoped. Of the roughly one in six patients with non-small cell lung cancer with adenocarcinoma and an EGFR mutation, nearly all will eventually develop resistance to treatment with EGFR inhibitors.

But Dr. Liu said what I needed to hear: We are prepared. We have a plan.

Dr. Liu asked if we would come back to Virginia. Yes! He indicated we didn't have to rush, maybe arrive in the next two or three weeks. We wanted to get home as soon as possible.

If you have a tumor, you want it dealt with yesterday.

In the meantime, the doctor would schedule a telehealth visit with a radiation oncologist on his team.

"I think in the short term, the answer is probably to do CyberKnife radiation in the L3 area," he said. "That's going to help with the pain, for sure. But it will also prevent the cancer from growing and causing problems in the surrounding nerves."

David and I now needed to get back to our home in Arlington. But first, I would get a cutting-edge blood test. Cancer sheds DNA and RNA into the blood. I would have what is called a *liquid biopsy* while in Palo Alto because it was not possible to perform a regular biopsy on the tumor in the bone area. The Guardant blood test would extract tumor DNA from my blood and hopefully find another mutation for which a targeted drug existed. Guardant sent a phlebotomist to Megan's house to draw my blood, so that the results would be ready by the time of my next meeting with Dr. Liu.

Everything Dr. Liu said that day was calming, reassuring. He's a master at explaining complex medical treatments in a way that a layperson can easily grasp, and that only enhanced our confidence in him.

He had a plan. He said it three different ways. "My hope was that we wouldn't be at this point yet, but we're ready for it," he said, wrapping up the call. "My hope is that this next treatment, this next adaptation will be the one that gives us that long-term control that we want."

It didn't. But it would take months to learn that.

I didn't remember this, but after we hung up and before David stopped the recorder, I began sobbing. I heard my tears at the end of our twenty-five-minute call. Again, we were faced with tough news to absorb. Each time there was a change for the worse, I experienced a mini grief. I always needed time to process, revive, charge forward. David, as usual, remained upbeat, feeling confident because there was a plan.

Later, I talked with Cutter and with Lydia, who both cried when I told them. That night, I sent an email to my inner circle with an update on my situation and our plans. It ended with the following:

I hate bringing you bad news that I know will upset you. But I hate even more that this is happening. I hope to follow the advice of our meditation instructor: "I'm trying to teach myself to not believe all my thoughts." As you all know, I have an incredibly public persona—except when it comes to my lung cancer. I'd ask you to talk about this only with people you need to share it with. I'm telling you everything I know now. No need to call with questions I can't answer. What I need most is your love and support. Yes, this sucks. Big time. But with the help of Dr. Liu and the Georgetown team, we will conquer the beast.

Phone calls became my bête noire. Friends would still call and ask a lot of questions, and I still had no answers. I knew their hearts were in the right place. Finally, I stooped to telling them to call David for updates.

We drove back to San Luis Obispo, packed up, shipped things home, Zoomed with our therapist, and managed to have all the kids come for a whirlwind visit before we bolted across the country. The radiation oncologist wanted us to fly, to get back as soon as we could. But COVID was raging. We decided to drive, agreeing that if I couldn't handle the car ride, David would drop me in Denver and I'd fly home.

On July 4, 2020, a Saturday, we headed east, keeping to the northern route, across states where COVID wasn't ravaging as hard. We were aiming to get home Wednesday night for a Thursday CT scan. The radiation oncologist and his team would take the data from the scan and draft a plan to feed into the highly sophisticated robot that would target my tumor down to the millimeter, zapping it with enough radiation to kill it without damaging nearby organs.

Our cross-country odyssey was something else. Even taking oxycodone every four hours and using an ice pack, the pain could take my breath away. David did the bulk of the driving, but I managed four or five hours a day.

By the second night, we had a routine. We checked into the hotel. David got gas while I walked, River. Then I put my gloves on and wiped down our room with Lysol. We ate from our cooler, which we packed each morning with hotel ice. At night, I made sandwiches for the next day. We ate only in the car or the hotel. We stopped only at designated rest stops. We stayed only at hotels that followed strict COVID protocols.

We made it home in five days, by which time I felt like someone was stabbing me with an electric knife. I wasn't always the nicest. David shone, he was so kind and patient. *How does anyone do cancer alone?* I thought.

To our surprise, David was allowed to come with me to the appointment despite COVID rules.

"I have good news," Dr. Liu said, as he walked into the examination room. The genetic blood testing revealed a new mutation, C797S. This mutation is detected in 10 to 19 percent of patients with Tagrisso resistance.

A year earlier, I'd read an article that said that if a patient was already on Tagrisso when they "progressed," there was no other targeted therapy available. But that was before 2020. Now doctors knew more about C797S. This showed how fast research was evolving with lung cancer.

The new plan was to add a drug called Iressa (Gefitinib) that "pairs well" with Tagrisso, said Dr. Liu. Tagrisso hadn't stopped working, but now I needed the Iressa to banish the rogue C797S mutation. Dr. Liu had one patient on this regimen, but the Dana-Farber Cancer Institute had treated many with this combination.

"Gefitinib (Iressa) plus Osimertinib (Tagrisso) is not a standard therapy," said Dr. Liu, "so yes, you could call this experimental."

Please let this experiment work, I thought.

Lucky for me, in addition to Tagrisso, AstraZeneca also made Iressa. I could continue to qualify, based on income, to receive both "miracle drugs" at no cost. Whenever I had to call AstraZeneca, before hanging up the representative would ask if there was anything else they could do.

"No," I'd say. "Thank you for saving my life."

In mid-July, I underwent three rounds of hour-long CyberKnife radiation treatments. Each time, a monstrous white CyberKnife robot moved over me like a friendly cartoonish giant, darting here and there, coming in close, pulling away, making no noise. I lay perfectly still on my back listening to R&B music on an old CD player while this robot moved in close, then skirted away. Given that they crank up the music and I'd taken a pain pill, it was a relaxing hour.

The radiation sapped my strength, and the two-drug combo caused diarrhea. I was weak and listless and sank into a depression during summer 2020.

It is completely understandable that you would feel the way you do now, texted my younger brother, Jay. *I think you're handling this incredibly well. I wish I could do something for you to make this an easier endeavor. And wish I could take some of this burden from you.*

For years, my only brother and I had lived fairly separate lives without a lot of communication. We were very close as children after our father died. But then I moved to the West Coast and went on our sailing trip for three years, and life has a way of taking you apart. Now that I was sick, however, he was there for me 100 percent. It felt good to be reconnected with him and his family.

A few months later, I was gobsmacked when I opened the CyberKnife bill. $114,981.94! Insanity. Yet I was fortunate enough to be well insured. With Medicare and a supplemental plan, I paid $780. (Note to others: Don't get cancer until you are sixty-five!)

I know the astronomical bill is meaningless, but it symbolizes everything wrong with our health care system and why so many are forced to declare bankruptcy over medical bills. What if I had to fork over that much money? I'd have to sell my house. I kept the bill as a souvenir, a reminder of how fortunate I am, and as a wish that all patients could have the same benefits.

Cutter was living in DC again, but because of the pandemic, he couldn't come inside our house. He brought me food and forced me to walk, first around the block, then farther and farther. My ennui lasted for a month, and by early September, I was walking four to five miles a day, sometimes up hills. I got back on a bike and started working out virtually twice a week with a trainer for thirty minutes. I was getting better, and for that and so much more, I was grateful.

However, I still had my off times. Since the return of the beast, I'd been participating in a weekly online support group called *EGFR Resisters*. I found it encouraging because the women who showed up were doing well. In mid-September, though, a woman appeared on screen, in bedclothes, unable to sit up. She was bald. Her treatment wasn't working. I am ashamed to admit that I found her story so unsettling that I muted her and walked away from the screen. It was hard to look at her and not picture my future. This was my third support group, and it was too much. I didn't return to the group.

I couldn't let my life be defined by cancer.

18

Dog No. 1

I adopted our dog, River, from a shelter in West Virginia. On January 6, 2021, the day Trump loyalists violently stormed the Capitol, the vet called us at 9:00 p.m. David and I unglued ourselves from the TV and I answered. We were waiting for the results of a tissue biopsy River had undergone from a tumor removed from his lip. No doctor calls you at 9:00 p.m. with good news. I steeled myself for the results. He made polite conversation, asking how I was.

"Depends on why you are calling. I'm guessing the news isn't good," I said.

The foul-smelling tumor on River's lip was oral malignant melanoma—within the same family of melanoma that David had had. It is very common in dogs older than ten years of age (River was fourteen at the time of diagnosis) and aggressive; if we did nothing, River would likely live three months. Now we all had cancer! We were a cancer cluster. My first instinct was to laugh. When we later mentioned River's diagnosis at our monthly melanoma support group, someone asked sardonically whether River might join the group.

David took the phone and peppered the vet with questions about immunotherapy, asking if there were trials in the area. He was already feeling a special kinship with River, given that he and the dog shared the same disease. The vet, who knew little about immunotherapy, was surprised by the depth of David's knowledge and promised to send us the names of vet oncologists. He suggested we meet with one to get a chest X-ray and an ultrasound to see if the cancer had spread. He mentioned chemotherapy, radiation, surgery.

David was keener to see if we could find nearby immunotherapy trials. Given most large dogs' life spans, regardless of the melanoma diagnosis, I needed to be realistic. River wasn't going to be around much longer. River was devoted to me, and I to him. He slept at the foot of our bed every night. He followed me from room to room. Wherever I was, he wanted to be. If I wasn't around, he'd follow David. He was a herding dog and was most happy when the three of us were together.

During the day, should I need to dash upstairs for a forgotten item, I talked to him the entire time, telling him I would be right back. Stay—do not carry that arthritic body up the steps for no reason. Like most dog owners, the four-footed love of my life owned my heart. If the existing treatments held little promise, I kept asking the vet, "To what end?" Why should we torture River with chemo or radiation if they weren't going to make him better? Or pay $475 for more tests and to see if it had spread?

I turned to Dr. Google to look up dogs, immunotherapy, and melanoma. According to the American Veterinary Medical Association, almost half of dogs older than the age of ten will develop cancer. I also discovered a 2019 study on dogs with mucosal or oral melanoma that backed up our vet's negative prognosis.

Biologically, we have much in common with dogs, and because of the similarities, treatments that work in humans sometimes work in dogs or vice versa.

"Genetically, you are a lot more like your dog than that mouse running around a cage in the lab," said Nicola J. Mason, an associate professor of medicine and pathobiology at the University of Pennsylvania vet school. "Where dogs really stand out is in the way they generate tumors and react to treatments, which is a lot like people."

Dogs are good test subjects because they develop cancer naturally—as opposed to inducing cancer cells in mice for experiments. Certain breeds are more likely to develop certain cancers. Lymphoma is more likely to affect golden retrievers, whereas brain cancer appears most often in Boston terriers, boxers, and bulldogs. Black poodles are prone to squamous cell carcinoma. Scotties, Westies, and Shelties are twenty times more likely to get bladder cancer than other dogs.

Immunotherapy worked so well in dogs with osteosarcoma that clinical trials were started to see if it worked in children with the same cancer. One of immunotherapy's first clinical milestones occurred in dogs. In 1999, Dr. Jedd Wolchok, an immunotherapy pioneer at Sloan Kettering, got funding from the Cancer Research Institute to investigate a vaccine for humans with melanoma. The trial stalled for logistical reasons, so Wolchok decided to try advancing the science by testing the vaccine on dogs. He teamed up with another cancer center to start a vaccine clinical trial in dogs. From 2000 to 2007, they tested the vaccine on about five hundred dogs. They found the vaccine increased survival when compared to surgery alone.

In 2010, ONCEPT became the first approved vaccine for dogs. Months later, an immunotherapy vaccine was approved for people with prostate cancer. The success of the animal trials had sped up the approval process for the human vaccine.

River's cancer hit me hard. Around New Year's Eve, shortly after River's tumor was removed, I had begun experiencing uncontrollable anxiety. My body thrummed 24/7. I couldn't drink my beloved morning latte; it only heightened my anxiety. I couldn't sit still. I couldn't concentrate. If I was sitting down, my foot tapped as though I were on speed. I often felt dizzy, causing me to worry that my cancer had morphed into leptomeningeal disease, another form of lung cancer that lives in the spinal fluid and brain. To get to sleep, I had to pop a Xanax and a melatonin tablet. Exercise was the only thing that helped. The faster I hiked, the steeper the hill, the more the anxiety eased. But as soon as I stopped, it was back. *You didn't fool me*, it would say. *I'm still here*. My subconscious was torturing me.

I had no idea what was triggering this. Just before Christmas, I'd been scanned every which way, and the results had indicated that all was good. So it wasn't that. It took my psychiatrist, someone I'd seen on and off since my diagnosis in 2019, to connect the dots: I was grieving River's impending death, but his cancer was also triggering my fears of my own illness, of suffering, of dying, of knowing the end was near. My anxiety didn't go away after talking to my psychiatrist, but hearing him say that my feelings made sense helped calm me.

He prescribed an antianxiety drug, Buspar, which I tried for a week. But gradually, as I threw myself into researching a drug trial for River, the anxiety disappeared almost as quickly as it had come. Perhaps the promise of prolonging River's life was intertwined with the hope of prolonging my own. Perhaps it was simply that I found a way to take control or at least to establish an illusion of control. Either way, I tossed the medication.

I found an immunotherapy trial at the University of Pennsylvania on the internet. I peppered Penn's vet nurse with the same questions we'd asked about David's trial. What was involved? How long was the trial? What were the side effects? And how did they treat them?

Turns out the treatments and their side effects are the same: steroids to reduce inflammation if the lungs or colon get inflamed. The nurse estimated we'd be getting between $5,000 and $10,000 worth of tests and treatment to determine the safety and efficacy of a new immunotherapy drug. Just as with David, the goal of immunotherapy is to reactivate a dog's own immune cells to attack the melanoma tumor as well as go after cancer cells in the rest of the body.

After we filled out all the consent forms, River was enrolled in the study. He would receive something called a STING agonist, which stimulates T cells and has caused tumor shrinkage in mouse models of cancer. A similar drug is being evaluated in human trials.

When the researcher asked us to give River a Trazodone pill two hours before his treatments, I *did* laugh. Trazodone was what my oncologist prescribed for *me* to quell my anxiety. It didn't work for me and, it turns out, it didn't work well for River.

When I explained to the Penn vet that she wasn't dealing with immunotherapy newbies, she said, "I'm sorry you had to go through that and now this."

Me too, but since David's results were so outstanding, we had high hopes for River. At the very least, he'd be contributing to science.

She still needed to walk us through trial risks. "The real risks are the side effects," said the doctor. "You are probably going to be very familiar with them. Anytime you stimulate the immune system, you have a risk of stimulating it too much. I feel like I have to explain it. I know you know, unfortunately. I think it's very unlikely in River's case."

River would get a five-minute injection of the study drug through a catheter. He was dog No. 1 in the trial. He would be the first of up to twenty dogs in the yearlong trial.

David and I drove River to Philadelphia six times in January and February 2021. We found a dog-friendly hotel in the heart of Philadelphia. We'd drop River off in the morning for treatment and testing, and we'd explore the surroundings. Each visit turned out to be a nice little romantic COVID getaway, especially seeing the famous Barnes collection of Impressionist and Postimpressionist paintings.

River got an extra year from the trial medicine, which was a gift. That October, we took him for a checkup and to get some pain medicine at our local vet. We'd been taking him to this animal clinic so often we rarely saw the same doctor. To our surprise, the vet who did the oral tumor surgery months earlier walked in. He was shocked to see River still alive and said so. River had even walked the mile to the vet and the same for the return.

But River really didn't have much longer to live. The next month, he couldn't walk up the stairs and was having accidents around the house. He no longer jumped up and greeted us at the door. We had plans to go to Los Angeles for a busy trip for Christmas, staying with three different family members. We were at that limbo point. Should we put him down now? It's one of the hardest decisions a dog owner will have to make. We just weren't ready. Instead, we found a wonderful caretaker who we knew would take good care of our boy.

We returned home to find River was moving at an even slower pace. It was time. Penn had asked us to bring him there so they could put him to sleep and later do an autopsy. Just before we were leaving to make the drive, David and Cutter got into an unusual screaming fight.

David had been up early cleaning up River's accidents in the house and getting the car ready for the trip. Cutter woke up just as it was time to leave. David assumed we were putting River in the car, but when he dashed out of the door, River was sitting on the steps and the door accidentally hit him and knocked him down the stairs. David was angry that River hadn't been put in the car and he stepped over him with the load he was carrying. Cutter exploded with anger.

"I've never seen anyone do that to an animal!" he yelled.

I knew what was behind it, and it had nothing to do with whatever they were fighting about—like many fights. It reminded me of a gigantic fight Judy and I got into while taking care of our dying mother. At this time, she was in hospice and a social worker stopped by.

I clearly recall the social worker saying, "Whatever you are fighting about, it's nothing. Your mother, someone you love very much, is going to die and there's nothing you can do about it."

It was the same with Cutter and David. We were taking our beloved dog of fifteen years to be put to sleep. This time, it was a one-way trip. Cutter had made him a steak dinner the night before.

Driving up to Pennsylvania, we told favorite River stories while Cutter and I took turns snuggling with River in the back seat. My favorite River story was when he took the elevator—by himself. Since he was so obedient, I usually walked down the hall of our seventh-floor apartment with him off leash. I instructed him to wait there and ran back to our apartment to get something. Returning to the elevator, my cell phone buzzed.

"Do you have a dog named River?" said someone who had read his collar with his name and contact number.

"Yeah, I do, why?"

"Well, he apparently took the elevator and he's wandering around the lobby saying hello like he's the mayor of the building," said the voice.

Apparently when the elevator doors opened, River got on, unleashed. Fortunately, he's a friendly dog.

River died on January 26, 2022. While we told River stories on the way up, we drove home in noticeable, heavy silence.

Two months later, Penn sent a thank-you letter and a small redwood box with River's ashes and name on it, and, as promised, his autopsy report. From Penn:

I wanted to check in to see how you've been doing since having to say goodbye to River. I also received the results of his autopsy report and wanted to pass along the findings: Melanoma was found to have spread to the lungs, mediastinum (area in the center of chest between the lungs), pancreas, left adrenal gland, and brain.

Other findings included a second type of tumor at the base of the brain (pituitary macroadenoma) that can cause Cushing's disease and a third, likely benign, tumor in the tonsil (plasma cell tumor). I don't suspect either of these likely contributed to River's decline in a substantial way.

The melanoma certainly acted increasingly aggressive toward the end. Thank you for letting us be a part of his journey—he was truly a sweet dog and the perfect first clinical trial patient (we have now treated ten dogs in the trial River kicked off). I promise to continue to research and (hopefully) find ways to improve our treatment of melanoma throughout my career.

19

Whack the Mole

My life as a patient with cancer became a game of whack-a-mole. One thing popped up, we attacked it, and then another appeared. That evolved into my pattern. But if I had learned anything, it was that every cancer is different. I couldn't predict my path, and neither could my doctor. In my support group, we may as well all have had different cancers, because no two of our diseases manifested similarly and our responses to treatments varied greatly.

In February 2021, while we were distracted by River's cancer, my own scans showed a tumor in my left lung. While all the other tumors were shrinking, this one looked to be growing, albeit slowly. Dr. Liu said that some oncologists might let it go, as the growth was in millimeters, and just keep an eye on it. But he wanted to be more aggressive. He was concerned that the beast might have morphed into small cell or squamous cell lung cancer—a whole different and, worse, ball game.

For the first eighteen months after my diagnosis, I lived like I didn't have cancer, swallowing a pill at night, offering a prayer of thanks to AstraZeneca and all the trial participants who had made it possible for me to live. I had dodged a bullet. I had lung cancer, but it didn't impinge on my life in any meaningful way.

That period of grace ended in summer 2020, when the cancer reappeared much sooner than my doctor or I had expected. Our hope had been that the CyberKnife radiation and the addition of a new drug to my regimen would tide me over for a few years.

Here I was again, less than a year later, facing my worst fears. But to my relief, the biopsy showed that the tumor was not small cell lung cancer. I had five more rounds of CyberKnife radiation to kill the growing tumor in my left lung. Whack that mole.

David and I planned a three-week trip to Alaska in August of that year. I knew I was fortunate—a lot of people couldn't dream of such a journey. But I was also scared. Of whether I'd be healthy enough to make it. Of what might pop up unexpectedly with my lung cancer to prevent me from going on the trip.

A month before our departure, scans showed more spots on my brain. Dr. Liu decided to double the amount of my Tagrisso and continue Iressa, which was doing a good job of controlling the C797S mutation I was also fighting. But since every patient with my specific lung cancer is different, he didn't know what to expect.

Still, our spirits were high when David and I set out on the Alaska adventure. We spared no expense: flying first class across the country, then a private cabin with a window for the ferry trip from Washington state to Juneau, and finally on to Anchorage, where we embarked on a spectacular trip past towering glaciers to the outer islands. From there, up to Denali, the highest peak in North America, where we hiked and hoped to run into moose. It had been my dream for thirty years to see a moose in the wild.

While in Anchorage, we rented bikes and went riding outside the city. Suddenly, it happened. People were stopped on the bike trail. We stopped, too. Not far away, there were two bull moose calmly eating near the trail. I couldn't get off my bike fast enough. I started taking pictures and crept closer until I stood just twenty feet away from a majestic moose with large, shovel-shaped antlers. It was potentially dangerous, but this kind of danger had never stopped me much. I was elated.

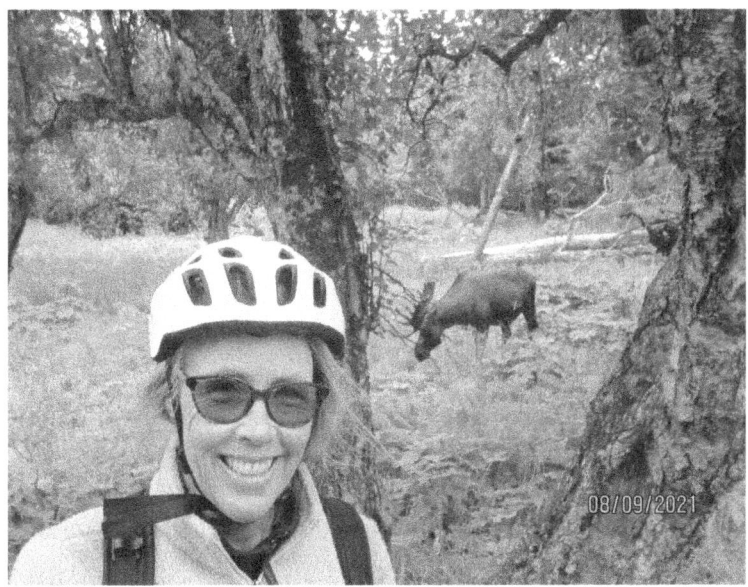

My favorite photo from our trip to Alaska is of this giant wild moose casually crossing the bike path. I made David stop so I could take a thousand photos.

As we neared the end of our journey, I started having a hard time breathing. I blamed it on the altitude. That might have been the case when I experienced breathing problems at the Grand Canyon rim, but the altitude of the national park we were exploring in Alaska was less than two thousand feet.

On the last hike of the trip, we walked up a hill on bouncy tundra. A guy, who must have been in his eighties, and I trudged up the hill together, stopping often to catch our breath. I had no idea why I was getting more and more winded.

By the time we got back to Anchorage, I could no longer pull my suitcase or carry my backpack. But I am one determined woman, and I wanted to attend the Alaska State Fair and see the giant vegetables that grow many times their normal size because of the nearly twenty-four hours of sunlight in the summer. Unfortunately, after a fifty-mile

Uber ride to Palmer, we learned that the vegetables would not be displayed until the following week.

Preparing to leave Anchorage, I was sick and nauseous. David dragged all our luggage to our early-morning flight. We had aisle seats in the back of the plane. I immediately grabbed the barf bag and began to fill it.

We were flying to San Francisco to see Billy and Laurence before their baby was due. We stayed at Lydia's flat not far away from them. I was feeling so poorly that I slept while David spent time with them.

Even though we were vaccinated, COVID remained a real threat. Plans were canceled with friends for fear I might have it. We finally found a clinic that was open and went there to be tested. The results the next day proved we were free from COVID.

Venturing out, I struggled to walk up the stairs to Billy's condo. Take a break, catch breath, continue. It was unusual for me to pause like that. But I was determined to have fun. Billy was trying to make us guess the two baby names they had decided on for their little boy. One option was Finn, and Billy tried to act like a shark. It hurt to laugh so much.

As I continued to feel ill and breathless, I reached out to Dr. Liu. He emailed me that there were four possibilities: a blood clot in my lung, COVID, the cancer, or pneumonitis. By the time we got home to Virginia, we dropped our bags and went to sleep.

The next day, we threw on shorts and sandals and went to see Dr. Liu. My oxygen level was so dangerously low that I was put on supplemental oxygen and wheeled to the emergency department, which doubled as a holding tank for patients with COVID. It was packed. People were lying on stretchers in the hallways as nurses and doctors scurried around, with families begging to see a doctor.

This was summer 2021. It was easy to get a COVID vaccine anywhere. Yet there was misinformation that the vaccine was going to make the young infertile or that the government was secretly planting microchips to track people or other nonsense. That meant that many of the hospital beds were filled with people who also happened to be unvaccinated. It infuriated the nurses to have to take care of patients with COVID who would not need a bed if they had been vaccinated.

I was taken to get a CT scan, which revealed a flaring case of pneumonitis in my left lung. Apparently, the drug cocktail was too much for my body, and I developed a lung inflammation, which was causing my breathing problems. Pneumonitis can be a side effect of several cancer treatments, including targeted therapies.

After the scan, I was fortunate to be put into a side room in the ER, and there we stayed, exhausted and hungry, for twenty-two hours, until a hospital room opened. Out in the hallways, people on stretchers were screaming for help. David waited most of the time with me, scrounging food out of vending machines and searching the hospital for sandwiches and drinks. I settled on a Snickers bar, thinking there was protein in the peanuts! A nurse finally found us two bland turkey sandwiches, but it was food and delicious.

Finally, I was taken to the ICU—not because I needed to be there but because that's where there was an available bed. My medications were halted. My condition really shook Dr. Liu.

"I did this to you," he said.

He was trying to reassure me that I had done nothing wrong. The treatment just hadn't worked as we hoped it would. It wasn't his fault, he was just doing his best as a doctor, but he felt responsible. He came to see me every few days while I was given steroids and antibiotics.

I spent nearly two weeks in the hospital—the longest I had ever been in one. I was tethered to oxygen, medication, and saline solution to keep me hydrated. A nurse had to get me up and on a portable toilet next to my bed, which wasn't easy because of all the tubes. The nurse did show me a nifty gadget that I thought I needed to buy for myself. It was about the size of a tampon and fit between your legs. All I had to do was pee on it, and liquid would get sucked up. It was a miracle for me. Might it save me from my many trips to the bathroom in the middle of the night at home?

I was eventually moved to a floor with regular patients and would walk the halls for exercise holding onto a nurse's assistant. I wasn't going home until my oxygen levels were higher, and neither was I going home without a portable oxygen tank.

The drugs I had been taking were not stopping the progression of the cancer. Dr. Liu wanted me to start a new chemo drug named Pemexetred (Alimpta), and I received my first infusion in the hospital. I finally went home in mid-September, hopped up on steroids to reduce the inflammation in my lung. I was so jittery that my leg was bouncing like a metronome.

I now considered myself a full-time patient with cancer. I would start on a mild chemo regimen where I would not lose my hair and would still be able to be active and ride my bike.

At first, I felt pretty good. After my second infusion, David and I drove several hours to the beach in Rehoboth, Delaware, where we biked twenty miles in the late-summer sun with our friends Cathy and Paul. That turned out to be too much. I would soon learn that I would become more tired with each infusion; the effect was cumulative.

Late in October, I was putting on my hiking boots, sitting on the edge of our bed. I was late to meet my friend Tara, and I didn't expect what was coming.

David sat down next to me and said, "I think we should get married!"

No down on one knee, no ring. It was as if he'd said, "I think we should go to the movies tonight."

I looked at him in shock. I'd been wanting to get married for years, but he wasn't interested, given this would be his third marriage, so I lost interest. "Why now?" I asked.

"I don't know, it just feels right," he said.

I said I'd have to think about it. We'd been together for ten years. We'd gone this long without getting married, what was the point?

David wanted there to be a record of our relationship. He thought we'd been through a lot together and had made a real commitment. This would be a way of showing that. He hadn't seen value in formalizing the relationship previously, but now he wanted the record to indicate we were together. He admitted he hadn't handled the proposal in a very romantic way; it was just the way he processed his thoughts.

The more I thought about our plans to spend time with all our kids in California that Christmas, the more I warmed to the idea of an intimate celebration with family.

We arrived in Los Angeles to cold and rainy weather. I was exhausted and took every chance to nap. We spent Christmas morning with family and New Year's with our good friends Judy and Roger.

Meanwhile, our kids were putting together our ceremony. They had offered to take care of everything—the flowers, drinks, location, food, even the vows. All we had to do was show up. We had always wanted our kids to be connected and close to each other, and in this magical moment, the people we loved came together to celebrate us as a family.

On December 28, 2021, we drove to Lydia's house. I was ushered upstairs where Joanna, Ted's fiancée, did my makeup and hair. I didn't have a wedding dress, but I had brought a three-quarter-length jacket an Afghan tailor had made for me.

Then the music started, and Lydia's kids—Carter, seven, and Baily, four—threw pink flower petals in front of me as I descended the stairs. Out on the patio waited David, his two sons, Ted and Billy, my son, Cutter, and Lydia. Billy's wife, Laurence, and their infant son, Finn, were there, along with Ted's fiancée, Joanna, and Lydia's husband, Andrew. Diana was on Skype from Miami, where she was visiting her family. It was perfect.

I knew we would pay for it when close friends and families asked why they weren't included. We'd just have to deal with that later.

In my usual style, I had given everyone a prompt: Why do you think this wedding was a good idea?

Billy spoke first. "We are gathered here to celebrate the communion of Dave and Lisa in what has to be the most spontaneous wedding that I've ever been a part of. I think this went about thirty-six hours from idea to reality, which is pretty impressive," he said.

He went on to say that in the beginning, our relationship wasn't easy—in fact, "Lisa and Dad have the honor of being part of the two most awkward moments of my life," he said.

We all laughed. But over the years, he continued, he had learned from us that adversity could be a gift, and that life was a journey.

Laurence, who got up to speak holding Finn like a baby koala on her chest, said that as far as she was concerned, we were already married. She and Billy had been looking at traditional wedding vows as they were writing the vows for this ceremony, and she realized we were already doing everything they said—supporting each other in sickness and health, trusting each other, building a new extended family. "I personally already feel like I'm your daughter," she said. "Regardless of whether you were getting married or not, Lisa, Finn was going to be calling you Grandma Lady, so sorry to break it to you, but that was already the plan."

Joanna, not much for public speaking, read a beautiful poem.

Lydia talked about how she liked the way David helped me find balance—how he supported me in having the adventures I wanted to have, while also insisting I have downtime. "And I am inspired by your gratitude," she said to me. "The other day we were talking and you said that instead of preparing for battle, you're asking your body for strength, and that you say thank you to it every day, and I thought that was so cool. You mean the world to me," she went on, and then had to stop because she was crying.

Cutter said that the main reason he thought us getting married was a good idea was that David and I laughed so much together, and as a certified mama's boy it, made him happy to see his mom smile that often. "And you're both full of courage," he said, and as he spoke the word *courage*, his voice broke, too. My eyes filled. For a moment I saw him as a little boy with white-blond hair traveling the seas. I remembered the way everyone welcomed us when they saw him. At the time, I thought I was showing him the world, but the truth was, he was showing me. The thought of leaving him, Lydia, or any of these dear people gathered around me pierced my heart.

Ted said that we fought well (thank you, marriage counseling), and that even with the fighting, there was always respect and love underneath it. The word that came to mind when he thought of us was *together*.

"There's no doubt about it," he continued, "you two have been dealt difficult hands. But in the end, you have made the absolute capital-B Best out of it. Dad and Lisa, I love you both. Here's to a long and happy marriage."

We moved on to the vows they'd written for us.

Did we promise to keep our cool when the other one was driving and giving directions?

We did.

Did we promise to laugh, cry, dance like no one was watching? (Or in Dave's case, *attempt* to dance like no one was watching?) To support each other through life's joys and sorrows, and to cherish each day together?

We did.

Did everyone gathered there today, promise to love, and laugh, and support this couple?

They did!

We took photos, sat down to a delicious lunch, and then went for a hike, although I moved at a slow pace.

We made it official a few days later. Ted drove us up to the Spanish-style Santa Barbara courthouse. Afterward, we found a cozy place for lunch. In lieu of a honeymoon, I took a nap.

We were the luckiest unlucky couple. We were married!

20

When One Person in Your Boat Is Calm

Since my diagnosis, I've had about four good years for which I'm grateful. That means years of hiking long distances, biking, hiking out of the Grand Canyon, hiking nearly every inch of the state park Montana de Oro near San Luis Obispo, California, multiple trips to the West Coast, attending Billy and Laurence's wedding, exploring Alaska, and the thrill of seeing two wild moose! All with my love, David. All things that I wouldn't have been able to do without advances in treating modern lung cancer. In other words, I've been able to live a pretty normal, adventurous, active life. Which is all I ever wanted.

Summer 2022 was a turning point. In May, the doctors found that the EGFR had mutated to leptomeningeal disease in the brain. In July, my doctor told me that my non-small cell lung cancer had transformed into small cell lung cancer (SCLC) in the liver.

As I write this, I have two cancers. Only about 30 percent of my original type of cancer has the bad luck of transforming into SCLC. No one really knows why.

The standard treatment is chemotherapy. It involves infusions of a potent drug called *etoposide* for three days in a row every three weeks for four sessions. Since I was going to lose my hair, I decided to have a small party and cut most of it off. Eventually, all my hair gradually fell out in big clumps anyway. I also did something I would not recommend: I bought a $500 nonrefundable wig with my friend Cina. I still had hair then, but it turned out I only preferred warm, cozy caps. I wore the wig just two or three times!

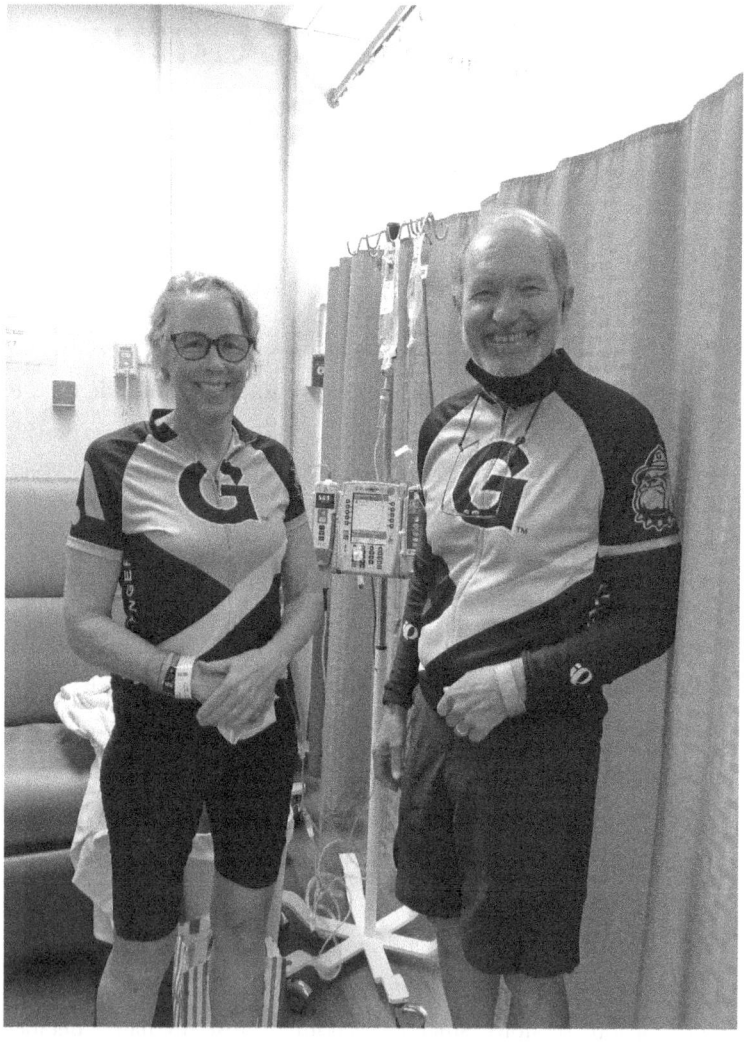

We proudly biked to my first chemotherapy treatment.

The etoposide treatment worked for only two months, so we tried another option called *lurbinectedin*. The FDA hadn't even approved its use until 2020, after my original diagnosis. Starting in December, I tried two cycles of lurbinectedin, which was also a painless infusion. This time my infusions were scheduled for only one day every three weeks.

Slowly I have recovered to a new base level that is lower than where I was before this new chemotherapy. The side effects are rough. I am losing appetite and losing a lot of weight. My energy is low, and I have reduced lung capacity. I am having trouble climbing the stairs at home, and getting up in the morning now is slow and arduous. I need to ask for more help—not a favorite thing—and David and I have decided to hire a home health aide to assist me and give David some needed time to decompress, exercise, and not feel locked in the house.

My neuropathy is getting worse, and I have stopped driving. I am sleeping more—a long stretch at night and a good nap during the afternoon. I am trying to protect time and energy every day to work on this book. David and I have our best time together in the early evenings, meditating, watching the news, talking.

The winter days are cold, and I wrap myself in extra sweaters. I have a favorite chair in the living room where I sit during the few good hours I have during the day.

I know that I am slowly dying.

"Will you miss me when I'm gone?" I ask David one night, overcome with the thought of leaving him.

"Enormously. Every single day."

"Will you miss me?" David asks me.

"I don't know," I say.

I don't know where I'm going. I don't know whether death is the end, dust to dust, or something I can't ever imagine.

It's hard to discuss with anyone. I cry at the thought of leaving the people I love, of them planning a memorial service, of the pain that lies ahead of me.

On Valentine's Day 2023, we see Dr. Liu to get the results after a CT scan of my abdomen. I wonder how many scans I've had. Probably fifty. I can tell right away that the lurbinectedin hasn't worked, just by his manner.

"I promised you from the start that I would always be straightforward," Dr. Liu says, leaning in toward me.

This must be the hardest part of being a doctor. I am glad David is sitting next to me. He takes my hand.

Dr. Liu says I have three options—none of them good. But we have to choose. No. 1 involves a different kind of chemo, which we all rule out—the chance of success is too low and the risk of more toxicity, including neuropathy, too high.

Nos. 2 and 3 are both more reasonable options. No. 2 involves immunotherapy, the wonder drug that tamed David's melanomas into disappearing. I know that immunotherapy works on SCLC sometimes, and it can work on mine—but I will have to stop taking Tagrisso, the medication that is treating my *other* cancer. Dr. Liu feels like Tagrisso is keeping things stable. Plus, there is only a small chance the immunotherapy will work. He floods us with information and percentages. I struggle to stay focused.

The third option is hospice. I am following my mother's footsteps. What would she think? She lived from January 1998 to September of the same year. I might go faster. Given my semi-addled brain, it is all I can do to understand.

Before we decide, I have a brain MRI scan to see if the Tagrisso is still working. I know the MRI drill well and hate the clanky, clumsy, whistle noises, sounding like pots banging while I lie in a white tube with my head locked into place with a catcher's mask.

"Don't move," the technician barks at me.

Hey, believe me, I don't want to do any part of this over. I lie perfectly still.

David sends out an email update to our family and friends explaining our difficult decision—immunotherapy or hospice, which I will do at home. He outlines the options in his note.

Immunotherapy has a 10-15 percent success rate in small cell lung cancer and a 5 percent chance of also helping the original non-small cell lung cancer. Success means eliminating the cancer for one to one-and-a-half years. However, taking it as an infusion one time every three weeks requires leaving the one daily medicine that has consistently worked in stabilizing the original non-small cell cancer—they don't work well together. Tough decision. Immunotherapy needs to start in two or three weeks to be helpful.

If we elect hospice, the small cell cancer could rapidly progress. Predicting how long it will take is impossible, but the doctor estimates one to two months. Knowing Lisa, I would guess closer to three to four months.

Cutter has been in western Massachusetts since January, directing his second feature film, and the last thing I want is for him to shut down the set and upend everyone's schedule. But I also want my baby at home to talk about the decision. I can't wait to see him. My brother gently lets him know to get home as quickly as possible. I wish Lydia lived closer.

Flowers from friends and family start arriving. One night my book club—arranged through David and my stalwart friend Jenn Weiss—come over and sing to me from our patio.

My brother, Jay, drives down from Connecticut to Virginia to visit several times. Again, I feel lucky to have him and his wife, Jeanna, and their four kids, who are equally loving, in my life. My brother still checks on me every day by text and visits often. I can't emphasize enough how loved I feel by my family and friends.

The day after the MRI, we have a tele-visit with Dr. Liu to get the brain results. They aren't good. The Tagrisso is no longer working, and the brain tumors are spreading. The cancer cells have migrated back to my cerebrospinal fluid.

Huddled up on our living room couch, David asks the critical question, "Does this change your thoughts about our choices?"

It does. It makes our decision much easier. With Tagrisso no longer working, trying immunotherapy without Tagrisso seems like a chance of success. I stop taking Tagrisso and start immunotherapy on March 2. Immunotherapy is a miracle treatment for some; not surprisingly, I want that for me.

When you are diagnosed with cancer, you go forward without a road map. Your life as you knew it is over. You're confused and terrified, suspended in time. The ground is always shifting. Should you really plan a trip to Alaska in a few months, or to Antarctica a year from now, when you are certain you're going to die soon? I always knew I had an incurable disease. I just didn't know when I'd run out of options. I postponed an $800 dental procedure after I was first diagnosed with leptomeningeal disease, which meant the cancer had spread to my brain. I was certain I was going to die, and it would be a waste of money.

Every day I walk a fine line between hope and reality. Hope that new treatments on the horizon will continue to allow me to live and to enjoy a full life, and the reality that lung cancer is by far the leading cause of cancer deaths in the United States.

There will always be something on the horizon that I'll question whether I should plan for. I try to live with that uncertainty by staying positive, appreciating the small moments, getting the most out of every day, and living a healthy lifestyle. I'm making peace with the possibility that my mother's omnipresent smoking caused my cancer. David and I continue to educate ourselves through support groups and reading so we can advocate effectively and together. We are a team. My successes and my setbacks are David's, and his are mine. But our stories are different.

It has been much harder to write the second half of this book, the half about my cancer. David's story has a beginning, a middle, and a very good end. According to his oncologist, the chances of his melanoma returning are in the single digits. I am not so lucky. David steadies me and keeps me optimistic. I need that.

As the Buddhist spiritual leader Thich Nhat Hanh says, "When one person in your boat is calm, the rest of the boat is calm."

David is that person for me. What if I were all alone?

We want our patients with cancer to be superheroes, brimming every day with optimism and resilience. I'll be honest: I'm not that superhero. Each day is a struggle, but it's also a gift, and I'm conscious of that in a way I never was before. When I climbed, huffing, to the top of a fire lookout in the middle of the Shenandoahs, the view was richer than it ever was, and when Lydia and her young kids came to visit, I made sure to enjoy every minute, despite the chaos.

In May 2023, Billy and Laurence are going to have a baby girl, a sister for Finn. David and I want to live long enough to be terrific grandparents.

As our friend Norm said to us at the beginning of our journey, "All you have to do with cancer is keep living. There are always new treatments on the horizon."

We live filled with hope and grateful for one more day.

Epilogue
David Marsden

As Lisa wrote in her last chapter, the summer of 2022 was a major turning point. I remember it too clearly. We were sitting in the garden of the Virginia Cancer Specialists building, a new circular structure surrounded by woods. Dr. Liu was trying to get us into an experimental program there. We had spent the morning talking to medical staff and now, on the patio outside, we were going through the pros and cons of the program. On the one hand, Dr. Liu was very positive about it. We'd had a good conversation the day before about Dr. Spira, who was running the trial, the effectiveness of the drugs, and how Lisa had a good chance of getting in. On the other hand, we weren't in the program yet; Dr. Liu wasn't sure if Lisa's brain cancer would disqualify her. And if she was accepted, we would lose Dr. Liu, whom we had come to trust and depend on.

We sat quietly, watching the wind blow in the trees. "What a different place to receive treatment than the university hospital," Lisa said. "I could get used to this."

"What did you think of the doctor?" I asked.

"I liked him. What did you think?"

Before I could answer, Carrie, who had led one of our support groups, appeared, seemingly out of nowhere.

"I'm so excited to see you joining this trial," she said, after she hugged us both and sat down. She was now working for Dr. Spira, she explained, and had seen Lisa's name on the schedule and had come out to find us. He was a terrific physician, she said. She liked working for him.

We chatted for a while and exchanged contact information. Lisa and I went home in excellent moods. It was as if the stars were aligning. This was the beginning of Lisa getting better—maybe even back to her old self.

The next day, we were on the porch at home when Lisa's phone rang. It was Dr. Liu.

"Hi!" Lisa said brightly, putting the phone on speaker so I could hear and we both could take notes.

Dr. Liu was quick and to the point. They had done a biopsy to make sure that they fully understood her current cancer. They'd found that the non-small cell lung cancer had transformed in her liver into a smaller and much more aggressive cancer.

Lisa exhaled audibly.

"It was unexpected, but pretty clear," Dr. Liu said. His voice was firm and grave.

I felt like I'd been punched—and hard. The conversation we'd had the day before was so upbeat! Dr. Liu had said Dr. Spira was great, the treatment sounded excellent, we knew one of the assistants... and now this. The experimental program was off the table.

I reached for Lisa's hand. She was shaking.

It wasn't so much that the new cancer was in the liver, Dr. Liu explained. It was that the cancer had turned itself into something completely different. And it required completely different treatment. Lisa would need chemotherapy.

"Everyone agrees on this plan," Dr. Liu said, referring to himself and Dr. Spira. "What I expect is a good response."

I was still reeling. For three and a half years, we'd been fighting a progressive cancer that was always changing and affecting different parts of the body. For three and a half years, we'd been finding solutions that seemed to be working. But now we were fighting a whole new animal. Now she'd have to receive the same treatment she'd watched her mother go through.

Lisa's eyes filled.

"Are the two cancers related?" I asked, stalling, giving her time to process.

In a way, Dr. Liu told us. The new cancer (SCLC) in the liver was a small cell variant. Although the larger cell cancer Lisa also had could be blocked by the Tagrisso she was taking, SCLC was different and could get around those blocks.

"It's a little more complicated now, Lisa," Dr. Liu continued, his voice getting softer. "We're treating more than one cancer at the same time, so we need to come up with a plan that really treats everything."

Lisa started to cry.

Dr. Liu continued to talk in a soft, measured tone. Even as I write this, I am impressed with how respectful and compassionate he was.

For this new cancer, he said now, the immediate first step was to start small cell chemotherapy. They would do four cycles and then go back to what she was doing now.

"Do I stop taking Tagrisso during chemo?" Lisa asked. I could see her trying to protect herself with research and facts. I also knew she was hoping she wouldn't have to give up the drug that had been helping her for years.

"Yes," Dr. Liu said. "This chemotherapy will kill the small cells and hopefully that's all we'll need." There were side effects, he continued— lower blood count, nausea, neuropathy, hair loss—but they'd help her get through them. The drug they used in this treatment was an old one, and a little more toxic, but it was the best.

"We'll get this under control, all right?" he said. "Responses occur very quickly with this."

Lisa was full-on sobbing. "I'm just having a hard time…" she said. It was hard for her to speak.

Both Dr. Liu and I were quiet.

She took a few deep breaths. "Why… are the drugs for small cell so old?"

Dr. Liu's voice softened again. "It is a hard cancer to study," he said. "A little less common. Nothing else we've developed has beaten it."

Lisa nodded, then picked up her pen.

We went over logistics. Dr. Liu had scheduled chemotherapy to start the following week. She'd have four cycles of treatments, each one lasting three days, with CT scans after the second and fourth cycle and an MRI at the end. Lisa had found her notepad and had begun to take notes.

"I know that this is the right treatment for us," he said again. "I'm optimistic about how well this is going to work."

"You are?" Lisa said, the same way she might have said, *Are you nuts?*

I almost laughed. She sounded like herself again.

"Yes," he said. "This is a chemotherapy that is very effective."

"Thank you," Lisa said, her voice breaking slightly. "I know you're not any happier than I am."

"I wish it were different, Lisa," he said. "But I know you're getting the right treatment."

We got off the phone and walked into the kitchen. We talked briefly about what had just happened, then we each went to our respective posts to carry out assignments. I started organizing notes, made a spreadsheet, and put everything on the calendar. Lisa took out her laptop and phone, making a list of who she was going to talk to and which appointments she would need.

The next thing I knew, she was on the phone with a friend whose daughter was a stylist to see if she could get a cut that would prepare her for hair loss.

This was the beginning of a physical decline that Lisa could not fully write about, even though she never stopped trying. So I hope to fill in some of how I remember those last few months.

Chemotherapy started in July. At first it wasn't so bad. We both rode our bikes to and from the treatments, and the symptoms, mainly nausea and neuropathy, were unpleasant but manageable.

By the second round of treatments, however, neuropathy in Lisa's feet made it hard for her to safely stop on the bike. After the first day, she drove and I rode my bike.

By the time she got to the third round of treatment, the neuropathy was so bad I drove her both ways.

By the end of the treatments, she had to put her bike away for good.

This was hard, but Lisa was Lisa. She had to stay active. Over the course of the last six months, we adjusted. When she couldn't bike anymore, she hiked. When she couldn't hike, she walked, even if it was just to the coffee shop, around the block, or to a local cemetery with beautiful views of the stars, where we'd often walked with River when he was still alive. (We tended to ignore the "No Dogs" sign. "Who can see that in the dark?" Lisa would say. "I can't. Come on, River. Just don't poop in here.")

As the fall progressed, however, she got slower, and by winter she needed to hold someone's arm or use a hiking pole. One morning in the last couple of months she said, "I can't. I'm just so tired." My heart sank.

That was so not Lisa, and it scared me to see her like that.

After that, walks got shorter, and she often would sit outside and talk to people. She always enjoyed watching the trees and the flowers and listening to the birds. I remember looking out the window one day and seeing her, sitting on the bench with a visiting friend, undoubtedly plying them with questions about their personal life, interrupting herself to say hi to someone walking their dog on the sidewalk, and thinking, *This is Lisa's soul.* Even when she could no longer travel the world, Lisa still wanted to explore it by asking people about themselves, gathering information for stories to share, and enjoying the natural beauty around her.

In December, Dr. Liu did a CT scan, plus another DNA blood test. The small cell cancer was already coming back. It was that fast. We had to start a completely different kind of chemo, more toxic, and with stronger side effects. The nausea, neuropathy, and hair loss got worse. Lisa got a wig, but she never really liked wearing it. The back spasms she had experienced all of her life became more frequent and lasted longer.

Right before Christmas, Lisa had another liver biopsy. It did not go well. Not only was the result the same (the cancer was back), but there were complications. She had internal bleeding at the biopsy site, which meant she had to stay in the hospital longer than expected. When she came home, she was in a lot of pain, which lasted for several days. Her back spasms were terrible, and she went for five days without a bowel movement while her liver recovered. We canceled a trip we were going to take to Asheville to see family.

"At least Cutter is coming for Christmas," Lisa said.

But when Cutter arrived, it turned out that he had COVID, so he had to quarantine.

It was the Christmas from hell. I was running all over town trying to find something for the constipation, or the back pain, or a way to change the drugs being prescribed, or a smoothie she would drink. Because of the neuropathy, she was having trouble getting up from the couch, and I almost pulled my back out helping her. When I went to the chiropractor to get relief for my back, he recommended I get forearm lifting straps, which I did. But I was burned out. It was becoming clear to me that we needed help.

After that, I started asking Lisa if we could get a caregiver to help me with cooking, cleaning, and laundry.

"I'm reluctant to have a stranger being around," she said at first.

Finally, though, she agreed to let me "research" it. It took time and joint interviews with more than one candidate, but we found a wonderful caregiver who was mature enough to understand that Lisa did not want her there, even if we needed her. She would follow my list of chores, then sit in the kitchen, just out of view, but not out of earshot. Lisa could call whenever she needed something.

For a few hours a week, I had time to run errands without worrying and even get in some exercise, mostly on my bike.

There were many ways we kept adapting to the new reality. Lisa needed blankets to stay warm, so wherever she was we had blankets. She set up a chair in the corner of the living room with cushions, a heating pad, and her laptop. She had a side table for drinks and food dishes, and a view of nearly all rooms and doors, so she could see who was coming and going.

For months after she passed away, no one, including me, dared sit in that chair.

She didn't have much of an appetite, so I tried to learn to cook for her. One day, I passed by her chair on my way to run an errand and noticed that she had only eaten half of her breakfast. I will certainly go down in family history as the person least interested in cooking, but I had worked hard to get her scrambled eggs just right. Two eggs with a little milk, some cheese, and not too dry. Add some fruit, toast, and yogurt, plus her morning coffee that I would have picked up from Starbucks the day before on my late-afternoon walk.

She saw me looking at her and the food and said, "Working on it."

My first thought was, *Not really*. Another time I might have said that out loud and she would have laughed or made some kind of a smart-ass reply, but that day I said nothing. She looked like she wanted to be left alone to research whatever burning question she wanted an answer to, so I left the house and went out to run some errands.

When I came back, the eggs were still there, cold.

"Lisa," I said. "Please try some of the eggs. You need the protein."

"I can't eat any more," she said tightly. "Do you want me to throw up?"

No, I thought. *I want you to get better. I want you to get strong enough to get up from this chair and get on a bike and ride around the city like we used to. I want you to appreciate the fact that I made those eggs. I want you to stop drifting farther away from me while I stand here, helpless.*

I took the plate and threw the eggs out. "How about a smoothie instead?" I asked.

Lisa was astounding in her ability to hold on. Until the very end, she was always aware of keeping her dignity and maintaining some control. In the last few weeks, her hair started growing back, and she was sure to mention it to anyone who stopped by.

She would take her hat off and point to the new growth and with a slight smile ask, "Did you see this?"

It was a way she could have something to show visitors, a distraction from the obvious negative physical changes, like that she couldn't get out of her chair to greet anyone because it was too difficult. When her cognitive skills began to fade, we shortened her visits with people, making sure that they were with her just long enough for her to present her best self.

She also didn't want anyone to pity her and was excellent at deflecting any attention put on her health.

If a visitor started the conversation with, "How are you doing?" she would quickly turn the conversation around by asking them how *they* were doing.

"I don't want to talk about me," she said when her West Coast best friend, Judy (I learned over time that Lisa had many best friends), came for a visit and asked how she was feeling. "I think about me all the time." She was sitting in her favorite chair, bolstered by pillows, which made her look a little stronger than she was. "Tell me about you. What is going on with your work?"

They spent the rest of the conversation talking about Judy and her work. Judy had to call me later, from California, to get all the information she wanted about Lisa's health and status.

Still, when everyone was gone, she would give in to how hard it was.

"Why me?" she would say. Or, "I think I am dying."

"Everyone is going to die," I would respond. "You just have a little more information than most."

She'd roll her eyes and ignore me. Finally, one day when I told her it was all going to be okay, she looked at me and said, "No, it is not. This hurts, and I wish it wasn't happening. Sometimes I just need you to listen."

That doesn't come naturally to me, to be honest. I spent most of my time trying to make things better, coming up with solutions, keeping myself busy to keep from getting upset. I didn't want to feel like things weren't okay. I didn't want her to suffer. I guess some part of me felt like if I could say or do the right thing, I could save her. But Lisa was never one for being saved. And she was also never one to be told to be happy or okay when she wasn't. So over time I learned to say nothing and let her feel whatever she needed to feel. She was never down for very long. She was amazingly resilient that way; it would only be a brief period before she'd be talking to friends or coming up with plans to visit the kids.

Eventually, I got better at listening. On one of our last walks when she said she thought she was going to die, I said, "What does it feel like?" to which she said, "Everything just hurts. Everything hurts so much."

By the beginning of February, her world—our world—got much smaller. We limited visitors as her energy decreased. One evening,

Lisa asked me to sit next to her on the couch after we had finished having dinner in the den. It was winter and the brick house was always a little cold downstairs. She was wearing her winter hat to stay warm.

Her laptop was open, as it often was, and she showed me a website called Five Wishes that she had been visiting. It asked questions—some she had answered, some not—about how she wanted to be treated medically, how she wanted to be remembered, and her memorial service. "This is what I want," she said. "Will you help me finish answering these?"

We worked our way through the unanswered questions one at a time. Some we treated like a business decision—"What does life support treatment mean to me?"—and others we treated almost as if we were planning a party.

"What kind of music do you want at your memorial service?"

"'Happy,' my favorite for dancing; 'R-E-S-P-E-C-T,' and..."—she paused as a song came on our streaming service—"... that one." It was, "Isn't She Lovely," by Stevie Wonder.

"Perfect," I said.

When it came to planning where the service would be, there was never any question that it would be outside in nature. The only discussion was where.

"This could get a little complicated depending on weather, restrooms, and parking," I said. She just stared at me, like, *Really?*

"I will handle it," I said.

"Let's talk to Amber," she said.

Amber was a niece who worked in a funeral home. Lisa ended up having a series of calls with her, which were extremely helpful. They went through the estate process, discussed specific details of the memorial service, down to the park bench where Lisa liked to sit.

"I remember laughing more than anything," Amber said to me later. "She handled it so gracefully."

They also talked through what would happen to her body after she died and came up with a few Plan B's. If Cutter was traveling, for example, did she want them to keep her body so he would be able to see her?

"That was a sad part for her," Amber remembered. "She said, 'Yes, keep me around.' But then she broke down and cried."

The hardest question wasn't on the Five Wishes list.

"What will you do when I am gone?" Lisa asked me more than once.

What was I supposed to say? "I will be okay, but I don't want to think about that," I'd say. "You're here now. Let's appreciate this."

After a while she filled in the answers.

"Don't get married again," she said when we were on a walk. "Take care of Cutter."

"If you do get married, don't get married quickly," she said, when we were falling asleep in bed.

I know she had similar conversations with other close friends and family.

It was a way of showing her love and support for those she cared most deeply about.

As the time got shorter, working on this book became very important. Although she'd been writing it alone, taking notes and crafting scenes for quite some time, in the beginning of 2023 she finally asked me to help even though she knew I did not enjoy it (almost at the level of my interest in cooking). We worked together on it from January to April, going over changes, talking through scenes and dialogue. At one point in the last few weeks, as I worked as a go-between with Lisa and her editors, we realized we really enjoyed working together.

"I wish we had discovered doing it this way earlier," Lisa said.

I did too.

Near the end, we made three visits to a weekend house in rural Virginia our friends Cathy and Paul owned. I would hike in the Shenandoah National Park and bike on the country roads while she stayed inside and wrote. It was a win-win.

It is the same quiet, peaceful, green setting where I have enjoyed finishing this in her absence. It seems the only place where I can work on it.

In March, Cutter returned home from shooting a movie in western Massachusetts. He took one look at my attempts at trying to feed Lisa and said, "I'll take care of getting calories in her. I know what to do."

"Great!" I said. *Good luck*, I thought.

But Cutter was terrific. He took smoothies to another level, somehow finding ways to get so many calories into each one that even the nutritionists were impressed. And I was grateful to have a partner. Somehow she kept eating until very near the end.

Overall, we slowly divided work and formed a team. Cutter took the lead on food and scheduling visits, while I worked on medicines and medical appointments. We both worked on encouraging exercise, which meant going for walks. We used a shared calendar to keep everyone informed. He was enormously helpful and he made me feel supported.

On one Wednesday night near the end of March, Cutter and I carried her upstairs after a visit with her friend Kelly, who now lived in Georgia (the country, not the US state) but happened to be passing through. Lisa's pain was worsening, and it seemed to be coming from several different places. Dr. Liu was doing what he could to increase her pain medication, but it clearly was not enough. I wanted to delay hospice as long as possible because I knew that once it started, the pain medication would mean we would lose contact with her. Cutter couldn't bear seeing his mom in so much agony. We had gone back and forth about this, but when she couldn't come downstairs that Thursday or Friday, Cutter and I agreed it was time. We discussed it together and then with Lisa, who agreed to go on hospice.

I was on hold with hospice in the living room when her friend Tara came downstairs and said, "I just talked to Lisa. She asked me what being on hospice meant and I told her it meant she was dying."

I froze.

"What did she say?" I asked.

"She nodded in agreement," Tara said.

I relaxed. I could never have said that to her, and I was so grateful to Tara for doing it. Somehow that helped reassure me we were doing the right thing.

That night I put Lisa to bed as I always did and helped her take her current pre-hospice pain meds. At this point, she was continually asking for more towels and more pillows. She was having some trouble breathing, which we thought was pain until the hospice nurse told us it was simply the cancer in her lungs. Still, it made her move around enough that she seemed uncomfortable. And it sounded rough, like something was blocking her lungs—which it was.

The nurse who had come to have us sign the electronic forms and assess the situation called me around 11:00 p.m. to take me through the new drugs that we'd need. I was too tired to enter them in my spreadsheets and went to bed.

As I started to get in bed, Lisa said, "Cutter," and pointed toward the guest room. I got Cutter and he, like I, thought it was just time to say good night. But she said, "Sleep here. And Diana."

I thought, *This could be interesting*, given the size of our two-person bed, but Cutter brought in a mattress for himself and Diana, and put it on the floor next to Lisa. He held her hand from her right side. I held her hand from her left. I think it was exactly the kind of situation she wanted. She was not in the hospital. She was with many of the people she loved, and everyone was together. In fact, it was exactly what she had requested in Five Wishes.

"I wish to have people with me when possible. I want someone to be with me when it seems that death may come at any time."

I know I fell asleep, and Lisa must have also because the next thing I knew, Cutter had come in with an air ventilator and the new prescription medicine. He had gotten it from an all-night pharmacy without telling anyone he was even gone. He also woke her up and had given her medicine without my knowing it. It was five in the morning. Lisa was still breathing, but it still sounded unusually gritty.

When I woke up again a few hours later, I was still tired. The night had been full of activities. Between Lisa asking for "help" for things we often had to interpret—towel? pillow?—and Cutter bringing new equipment, I had been in and out of sleep all night.

I looked at the medicine that Cutter had found. It was what I considered the "Goodbye Lisa medicine": a heavy dose of narcotic that would handle her pain, which we needed to do, but would also be the end of any meaningful conversations. I felt worn out and raw, like we had made another step on the staircase of goodbye. I accepted each step but didn't like any of them.

I had some friends meeting me on our porch that morning—I called them the Tea Timers since we used to meet for tea when we worked together. Lisa was always very supportive of me getting together with them. I whispered in her ear, "I'm going to go down and meet the Tea Timers, but I'm here if you need anything."

She did not respond, which was odd. Normally, I would have expected at least a squeeze of my hand. I noted this but went downstairs anyway, as Cutter and Diana were in the room with her and her breathing had not changed.

Out on the porch, I briefly told my friends what was happening, a *Reader's Digest* version, and then moved the conversation on to our usual topics: international affairs plus a splash of politics. It was so strange. When someone you love is dying, your world is so tiny. Time stops. You listen to every sound they make. And yet when you walk out the door, you see that other people's typical days are out there chugging along. On my street, couples walked by on the sidewalk with their dogs. A group of cyclists sped by, shouting to each other over their shoulders, as if nothing out of the ordinary was happening. As if it was just another pretty spring day. Part of me was happy for them. Part of me was happy for the distraction and the return to normalcy. And part of me felt guilty that I wasn't by Lisa's side.

Near the end of our meeting, I heard someone knock on the front door. It was the hospice nurse, there to check on Lisa and finish paperwork. "Come on in," I said. The Tea Timers left, and the nurse and I went upstairs where Cutter sat with Kelly, who was still visiting. Diana was on the phone, handling calls from other friends.

The nurse assessed Lisa and then started educating Cutter and me on the new medication. I asked for her to pause so I could get my notebook to take notes.

Cutter either said, "You don't need notes, Dave," or rolled his eyes, or I imagined him thinking, *Come on, Dave, you don't need notes now. We're all here listening*—I don't really remember. I do remember feeling like I had to explain myself for some reason, and then I broke down.

"I know my notes and lists are only helpful to me," I said. "But I need to stay organized. I can't..." For the first time, I started really crying.

Cutter came over and hugged me. I cried harder, and we stayed like that until I was done. When I opened my eyes, Lisa was looking at us. It is odd to say because I noticed no change in her expression—she was barely conscious—but somewhere I knew she loved that moment of seeing us together: Her two families blending as she had always wanted.

We went back to work learning how to administer the morphine. Diana and Kelly stayed next to Lisa, massaging her feet. Kelly was talking to her softly.

We were in the middle of discussing how to combine the medicines for pain and anti-anxiety when Kelly said, "I think she's stopped breathing."

Cutter and I raced to Lisa, Cutter on one side and me on the other, just as we had slept. I moved my hand up and down her cheek and let her know that it was okay for her to go, that she was loved and would be missed. She took another struggling breath or two, then… nothing.

The nurse listened to her heart. She took her wrist to check for her pulse.

"Yes," she said. "She's gone."

I didn't want to write this epilogue. I didn't want to write any of this book. I wanted my wife to live and finish it herself. That did not happen. But near the end, this project became an act of devotion between the two of us, a place where we could remember what we meant to each other, where we could tell each other our story, again and again.

And who doesn't love reliving their own love story? Especially as your love deepens and grows. Especially if you know one of you is going to leave.

Lisa knew the book wasn't done. Had she lived, there would have been at least another chapter and another draft and another draft.

Had she lived, we might have been able to convince her to put more romance in. To tell more about that night, I told her I loved her—which, I'm sorry to say, could only happen after she told me she loved me first.

But she didn't make it that long. She lost her energy, her ability to focus, and finally her ability to breathe. She worked on this book up until the very last day of her life, giving it every bit of her rapidly declining energy, even as the cancer affected her brain—even when all she could manage was a thumbs-up or a thumbs-down on a suggested edit.

Near the very end, she often lost the ability to complete a sentence, which left us guessing or asking her to clarify. The most painful sentence was, "I don't want to…"

We knew the missing word was *die*, and it hurt, even in its absence.

But here is what I know she'd want you to know: This is a book from someone who loved to tell a story and who loved connecting to people and helping them. It is about a late-in-life couple finding each other (yes, it *can* happen!). It is for patients with cancer and their caregivers experiencing the life-changing effect that a cancer diagnosis can have.

Lisa wanted to tell the truth. She wanted to help other patients with cancer and their caregivers. This is something we share. Her desire to research the details of our treatments sometimes led to her bringing her notes to our doctors' meetings and spending valuable time asking them questions. They were always generous and gave willingly. I continue to participate in support groups and offer my experience and learning as I can.

I feel lucky to be alive and so grateful for what we learned from our relationship. The most important lesson: Every day you are with the person you love is special, never to be taken for granted.

Recently, the therapist who helped us through both of our cancers told me how extraordinary it was to watch us work together as a team, shifting directions between being patients and caregivers. She felt it showed a profound strength and asked if I saw it as a strength. I did not. To me, Lisa was there for me, and I was there for her. I guess that is true love. We loved each other to the last minute we were together.

I love her still.

Just as helping Lisa finish her book and writing the epilogue has been hard, I now find finishing this project a challenge. The final words will be hers, but before I go, I have a couple of last stories to share.

On April Fools' Day 2012, as I was excited (and a little anxious) to prepare for a date with this woman I'd met on Match.com, I got a phone call. It turned out to be Lisa, who I'd never spoken to before on the phone.

She asked, "Is this some kind of an April Fools' joke? You were supposed to let me know where and when we plan to meet."

Apparently, the email I had sent was lost in cyberspace.

For the next eleven years, we had the ride of a lifetime. I never met anyone for whom living fully was more a part of who she was. She always wanted something new; she was always attracted to the edge of things that were exciting and different. In her kitchen on her refrigerator, she kept a sign with a quote from Winston Churchill: "Never, never, never give up." She lived that until the last day she was alive.

Lisa passed away on April 1, 2023, eleven years to the day after our first date.

There has been a profound emptiness in my days since she left.

I miss planning the next adventure. I miss how we'd start the day with a snuggle in bed and then make the bed together, after which we'd have a mandatory hug. I miss our evening ritual of listening to a meditation and picking a show to watch. Doing those little things myself reminds me each day that she's gone. And even now when I go to the doctor for a scan or for a checkup, I miss having her at my side. Yet somehow I feel like she still is.

I am so grateful for the time we had together. For years we'd known what the ending would be. We didn't know exactly when it would come, but we slowly learned to appreciate every day, and as the end became obvious, we became more grateful for every moment.

We learned how to love and lose and still enjoy the journey.

On March 31, 2023, I was helping her get into bed. At this point her ability to speak was rapidly declining, as was her energy. But as she lay down, she looked at me and said, "I love you so much."

I responded the way we both did, "I love you more."

It was our last full conversation.

I love you so much. I love you more.

We'd said it all. We used the time wisely. That was our goodbye.

Everyone Lisa mentioned in this memoir has been a hero to us. In addition, there are even more friends and family—not mentioned—who jumped in at different times and in so many ways that I could not even list them. Lisa's network of friends and family, as I have learned, seems endless. Their love and support in the form of food, flowers, cards, appropriate workout routines, and just talking about "something else" all contributed to make our journey better than it ever could have been on our own. To all of them, you have our heartfelt gratitude.

Lisa was also profoundly inspired by her doctors and all the health care workers who treat people with cancer, as well as the other patients who walked this path before or with her—especially those in clinical trials. She was in awe of their courage, strength, and spirit. She mentioned this nearly every day.

And now as promised, I will let Lisa have the last word. Before she died, she gave herself a writing prompt: "How do you want to be remembered?"

Her answer seems a perfect end to her memoir.

I want to be remembered as someone who grabbed life by the horns and lived it fully. I have spent my life seeking opportunities that have challenged me. I have taken risks that I am proud of. I am incredibly proud that Cutter's dad and I quit our jobs and spent three years sailing through the South Pacific, essentially retiring while we were young. It was the right thing to do. I would like it to be an example. I am equally proud of making the decision to follow love to Afghanistan and have the adventure of a lifetime with David. It was the right thing to do. Taking risks, no matter what, are how we live life to the fullest, and how we can learn so much about ourselves.

I want to be remembered as someone fun, lively, who loved life, and made wherever she was that much better and more fun because I was there. I have always taken seriously my mom's words, that if you accept an invitation, you assume an obligation. So wherever I've gone, I've wanted to make my being there something others enjoyed.

I want to be remembered as someone who loved strongly, lived fully, and cared so much for the people in my life, and hope I've added something of value to each of their lives. I want to be remembered as someone people thought of as compassionate and empathetic, who gave as much of herself as she could, and was a good, if not excellent friend, as my friends have been to me.

I want to be remembered as a good, loving mother to both Cutter and Lydia and as an example of how to live. She and Cutter have brought endless joy to me. I want them to take smart risks and not hesitate out of fear or convention.

I want to be remembered for my giveback game, for trying to do what I could to make the news industry more diverse.

I have tried to live my life as an example. No doubt, I have failed along the way. But throughout life, love for my family and for my friends guided me. For this, I will always be grateful.

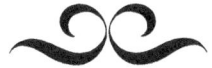

Appendix: Advice for Patients, Families, and Friends

Having been through two stage 4 cancers, David and I have learned a lot, and here are some things that may help others who are concerned about their health or have recently been diagnosed with cancer.

If you or someone close to you is worried, get it checked out.

When I saw a purplish lump on David's head, I pushed him to see a dermatologist. When I had a pesky, persistent cough that I wasn't too worried about, David pushed me to see a primary care doctor about it. I'm grateful to him for that and grateful that my doctor ordered a chest X-ray just three weeks after I'd first mentioned the cough to her. Far too many patients with lung cancer lose precious time as doctors wave off concerns—*It's an allergy, use an inhaler*—before finally ordering a chest X-ray. Listen to your loved ones, and don't be afraid to insist that something you're worried about be tested.

If you're diagnosed, seek out places where they are doing cutting-edge medicine.

If you have a stage 4 cancer, go straight to a comprehensive cancer center that is doing research, such as Georgetown or Dana-Farber.

Advances in cancer treatment are happening very fast. The GO2 Foundation for Lung Cancer and others report that 80 to 85 percent of patients with lung cancer are treated in the community hospital/medical setting. Community hospitals can be wonderful places, but they aren't going to be doing the cutting-edge medicine you need to treat a life-threatening cancer. At the very least, make sure you see a thoracic/lung cancer specialist. Same for melanoma. It's far more serious than anything your dermatologist can handle.

Be (a little bit) patient. Get a second and even a third opinion.

Getting a cancer diagnosis is terrifying. Nothing feels stable. There's a temptation—born out of fear—to go with the first doctor's recommendation. We get it. We want the treatment to start yesterday. But it's critical to gather as much information as possible before deciding. David and I saw several doctors for my cancer before deciding on Dr. Liu, and we learned a lot along the way. With David's cancer, we saw or sent records to five melanoma specialists. When you see a specialist, ask as many questions as you want. If they don't have the time to answer, they're the wrong doctor. It helped us to write down our questions before visits. And I keep a running list of questions and concerns between visits. When I see Dr. Liu, I hand him the list.

If a treatment plan involves surgery and medications, remember that this isn't a sprint.

Once home from the hospital, set up a spreadsheet or get a notebook to keep track of your medications: how much, when they are taken. Write it all down. And share it with other caretakers. We set up a special calendar after David's surgery with all his medical appointments.

Limit visitors. They can take a lot out of the patient, who feels the need to be "on." Once we got a rhythm going after David's surgery, our kids set up a schedule so that one of them was "on duty" each week to help me until we didn't need it anymore.

Set up a CaringBridge or something similar. All your loved ones will want to know what's going on and will have a boatload of questions and concerns. It can feel overwhelming to send separate updates to lots of different groups. We used CaringBridge to keep David's fans apprised of his progress. We posted updates and they were notified and knew where to go to learn the latest. Since I wanted more privacy, I kept a close circle updated. We are all different, and you can set up the information-sharing system you feel comfortable with.

Only listen to doctors who know your specific cancer.

When I got a bronchoscopy in March 2021, the radiation oncologist performing it told me that based on a new scan, it looked to him like the cancer had spread to my right lung. I passed three angst-ridden days waiting for the results, his words banging around in my head. In fact, the cancer hadn't changed; it was only inflammation. Lesson learned: Take information only from the oncologist who knows your disease inside and out. That doctor might have been the best at bronchoscopies, but he didn't know what he was talking about when it came to my cancer. Something identical happened with David when he ended up in the hospital on an Easter weekend. The ER doctor did a CT scan and concluded the immunotherapy wasn't working and that David's tumors were growing. They admitted David to the hospital. It wasn't until the next day when his oncologist was on duty and explained that David's tumors were *not* actually growing. Twice we made the same mistake, and it resulted in unnecessary worrying.

Keep a diary.

By doing so, you have references to how you might have felt a year ago, or a month ago, to report to your doctor. For example, when I had a tough round of three days of chemo every three days, it helped to know how it affected me after the first round and then after the fourth. It also documents how lousy you felt after some treatment, but that it got better. It helps you keep straight your treatments and can provide valuable information to your doctor. We also kept an ongoing list of questions for our doctors, so the day of the appointment we had our questions printed out and ready to go. Believe me, you will always have questions, so keeping a list provides answers.

Find the support you need and are nourished by and rely on it.

Family support is critical. Cancer doesn't just happen to one person; it affects a much larger circle of loved ones and friends. Involve your family if you can. Don't try to go it alone. At the very least, you need a "cancer partner"—a spouse, a son or daughter, a parent, or a friend. We formed an A-team with two of our research-oriented kids and three doctor friends. One of the doctors came to every appointment with me when I was first shopping for a specialist for lung cancer. David comes to all my appointments. Our kids often are on speakerphone. And—this is critical—always have your partner record the doctor visit (with their permission), or do it yourself if you're there alone. It's amazing how much more you get out of the visit when you listen to the recording later at home. There's always so much to absorb and particularly at the beginning when you're scared, you miss a lot—another reason why it's so important to bring someone with you.

David and I also find support groups very helpful. Find one that addresses your specific disease. But give yourself permission to pull back from it, too. There have been times I've needed to do that for my own emotional health. Too much focus on your disease can be debilitating.

Suggestions for friends of those diagnosed with cancer:

Don't ask a lot of questions when someone is newly diagnosed. We know you mean well, but your friend is stepping into a new universe and is as clueless as you are. When they come home from the hospital after surgery or treatment, send flowers or food or whatever you think will help, but give them time before visiting. Visitors mean well and are anxious to see their friend or loved one doing well, but visits are also very tiring. If you do visit, make it brief—even if your friend says, "No, stay longer." Don't ask if there's anything they need. Figure out what they need and offer to do it, whether it's walking their dog or

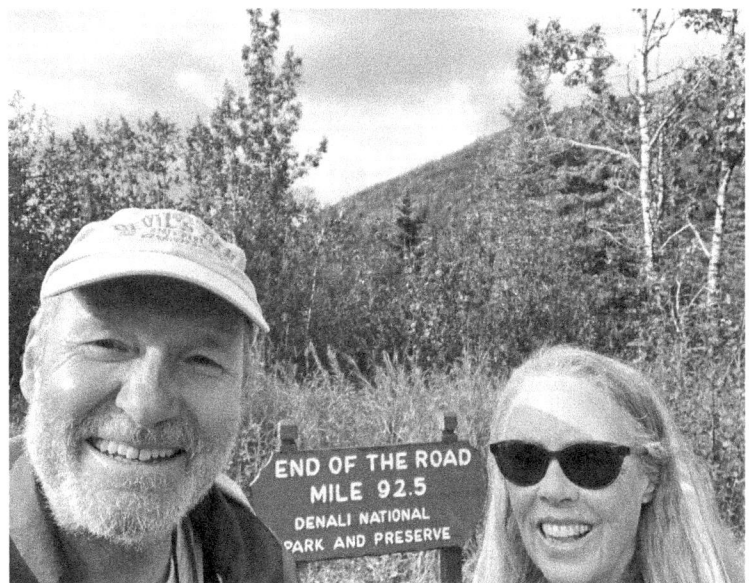

Near Mt. Denali in Alaska on what would be our final adventurous trip.

driving them to a medical appointment or cooking dinner. Try setting up a "dinner tree" (after you've checked for food allergies), where you coordinate among your friends who will drop off dinner on what night.

And finally....

While we all live with uncertainty, we patients with cancer live with a little more. I am ever so slowly learning to walk a damn fine line—trying to live well while dealing with a life-threatening disease. It's a tough, day-by-day balancing act, one I'm still navigating. Find whatever brings you some serenity or comfort: therapy, meditation, yoga, exercise, hikes, biking, acupuncture, lectures and conferences on your disease, education, or support groups. Do your best to thrive.

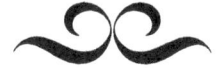

About the Author

Alicia (Lisa) Shepard was an award-winning journalist, professor, media trainer, media critic, and op-ed writer.

Shepard's extensive resume includes writing for *The New York Times*, *The Washington Post*, the *Los Angeles Times*, the *Chicago Tribune*, and *People* magazine. She is a former ombuds for National Public Radio and a contributor to *USA Today* and NBC News.com.

She was a longtime mentor/editor for the Op-Ed project, which teaches people whose voices are underrepresented in journalism how to publish opinion pieces. For years she volunteered each summer to teach students the basics of journalism for the Urban Journalism Workshop, sponsored by the Washington Association of Black Journalists.

Shepard was an expert on the lives of *Washington Post* reporters Bob Woodward and Carl Bernstein, who broke the stories on the Watergate break-in that led to the resignation of President Richard Nixon in the 1970s. She spent four years interviewing more than 175 people linked to Watergate for her 2006 book, *Woodward and Bernstein: Life in the Shadow of Watergate*.

She also coauthored the book, *Running Toward Danger: Stories Behind the Breaking News of 9/11*, about the challenges faced by journalists covering the 2001 attack, and in 2004 wrote *Narrowing the Gap: Military, Media and the Iraq War*.

For ten years, she wrote about ethics and the news industry for *American Journalism Review*, where she won awards for media criticism. For that work, the National Press Club awarded her its top media criticism prize three different years.

For many years she was judge on the National Press Club's Journalism Awards Committee, helping to select Grand Prize winners for the Robert F. Kennedy Book and Journalism Awards. In 2003, she was a Foster Distinguished Writer at Penn State University.

She taught media ethics, interviewing, and long-form writing at various universities including in the master's degree program at Georgetown University from 2007 to 2010. She also taught at American University and was a Times Mirror Visiting Professor at University of Texas at Austin from 2005 to 2006 where she taught a class on Watergate and the press. She was a visiting professor in 2012–2013 at the University of Nevada, Las Vegas, and at Cal Poly in San Luis Obispo, California, in 2020. In 2017, she was a Visiting Distinguished Professor of Ethics in Journalism at the University of Arkansas.

On a personal level, she sailed a thirty-two-foot sailboat with her son and her then-husband, through the South Pacific for three years. They cruised the islands, and she wrote about their adventures. They also spent two more years in Japan, where she learned to speak Japanese, wrote, and taught English. In 2002, she biked 517 miles from Amsterdam to Paris and in 2012 biked 502 miles across Iowa for RAGBRAI.

She was consistently curious about others and showed her love of adventure and courage by moving to Kabul, Afghanistan, in 2014. There she worked for two years with nonprofits and USAID, helping train Afghan journalists.

Shepard graduated from George Washington University with honors in English and received a master's degree in journalism from the University of Maryland in 2002. Her life and contributions to journalism were noted in obituaries and articles, including those published by *The New York Times*, *The Washington Post*, the News Literacy Project, and the Journalism and Women Symposium.

She is survived by her husband, David Marsden, a marketer formerly with USAID who brought this book to publication; her son, Cutter Hodierne, a Sundance-award-winning filmmaker; two stepsons, Ted and Billy Marsden; three grandchildren; a brother, J. Powers Shepard; and a half sister, Emily Riddell.